FAVORITE BRAND NAME

DIABETIC RECIPES

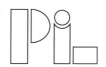

PUBLICATIONS INTERNATIONAL, LTD.

Recipe Development: Pam Eimers, Lisa Kobs, Karen Levin
Nutritional Analysis: Linda R. Yoakam, M.S., R.D., L.D.

Photography: Proffitt Photography, Chicago
Photographers: Laurie Proffitt, Cindy Trim
Photographers' Assistant: Pamela Callahan
Prop Stylist: Kathy Lapin
Food Stylists: Carol Smoler, Moisette Sintov McNerney
Assistant Food Stylist: Susie Skoog

Pictured on the front cover *(from top to bottom):* Key Lime Tart *(page 84),* Beef & Bean Burrito *(page 78).*

Pictured on the back cover *(clockwise from top left):* Greek Spinach-Cheese Rolls *(page 16),* Curried Chicken & Vegetables with Rice *(page 64)* and Mixed Berry Cheesecake *(page 82).*

ISBN: 0-7853-3459-9

Manufactured in U.S.A.

8 7 6 5 4 3 2 1

Nutritional Analysis: Nutritional information is given for the recipes in this publication. Each analysis is based on the food items in the ingredient list, except ingredients labeled as "optional" or "for garnish." When more than one ingredient choice is listed, the first ingredient is used for analysis. If a range for the amount of an ingredient is given, the nutritional analysis is based on the lowest amount. Foods offered as "serve with" suggestions are not included in the analysis unless otherwise stated.

Microwave Cooking: Microwave ovens vary in wattage. Use the cooking times as guidelines and check for doneness before adding more time.

FAVORITE BRAND NAME

DIABETIC RECIPES

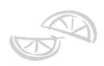

Facts About Diabetes

Low-calorie, low-fat, low-cholesterol and low-sodium—buzzwords of the decade and for a good reason. People today are more aware than ever before of the roles that diet and exercise play in maintaining a healthful lifestyle. For people with diabetes and their families, the positive impact good nutrition and physical activity have on well-being is very familiar.

Diabetes is a disease that affects the body's ability to use glucose as a source of fuel. When glucose is utilized improperly, it can build up in the bloodstream, creating higher than normal blood sugar levels. Left unchecked, elevated blood sugar levels may lead to the development of more serious long-term complications like blindness and heart and kidney disease.

Not all cases of diabetes are alike. In fact, the disease presents itself in two very distinct forms—Type I and Type II. Development of diabetes during childhood or adolescence is typical of Type I, or juvenile-onset, diabetes. These individuals are unable to make insulin, a hormone produced by the pancreas that moves glucose from the bloodstream into the body's cells, where it is used as a source of fuel. Daily injections of insulin, coupled with a balanced meal plan, are the focus of treatment.

People who develop Type II diabetes, the more common form of the disease, are typically over the age of 40 and obese. These individuals produce insulin but the amount is insufficient to meet their needs, or their excess weight renders the hormone incapable of adequately performing its functions. Treatment includes balanced eating, moderate weight loss, exercise and, in extreme cases, oral hypoglycemic agents or insulin injections.

Maximize Health, Minimize Complications

Diabetes increases one's risk of developing high blood pressure and high blood cholesterol levels. Over time, elevated levels may progress to more serious complications, including heart and kidney disease, stroke and hypertension. In fact, research shows that individuals with diabetes are nineteen times more likely to develop kidney disease and four times more likely to suffer from heart disease or a stroke than people who do not have diabetes. While heredity plays a major role in the development of these complications, regular check-ups with your physician and registered dietitian to fine-tune treatment strategies are good ways to help minimize complications. Strategies for treatment vary among individuals, yet overall goals remain the same: achieving and maintaining near-normal blood sugar levels by balancing food intake, insulin and activity; achieving optimal blood cholesterol levels; and improving overall health through good nutrition.

Balance is the Key

Achieving optimal nutrition often requires lifestyle changes to balance the intake of nutrients. The United States Department of Agriculture and the United States Department of Health and Human Services developed the Dietary Guidelines to simplify the basics of balanced eating and to help all individuals develop healthful eating plans. Several of the guidelines which follow were adjusted to include the revised 1994 American Diabetes Association's Nutrition Recommendations. Because these recommendations are broad, work with your physician and registered dietitian to personalize the guidelines to meet your specific needs.

Eat a variety of foods. Energy, protein, vitamins, minerals and fiber are essential for optimal health, but no one food contains them all. Including a wide range of foods in your diet and using fats sparingly are easy ways to consume all the nutrients your body needs. Carbohydrates should comprise between 45 and 55 percent of total calories and protein should contribute between 10 and 20 percent.

Maintain a healthy weight. Excess weight can worsen your diabetes and encourages the development of more severe complications. Research shows that shedding 10 to 20 pounds is enough to initiate positive results for obese individuals. Combining a healthful eating plan with physical activity outlined by your health care team is the best medicine for maintaining a healthy weight.

Choose a diet low in fat, saturated fat and cholesterol. Fat has more than double the calories of an equal amount of protein or carbohydrate. Thus, diets low in fat make it easier to maintain a desirable weight and decrease the likelihood of developing high blood cholesterol levels. Limit fat to no more than 30 percent of total calories, saturated fat to no more than 10 percent of total calories and daily cholesterol to no more than 300 mg. The 30 percent of calories from fat goal applies to a total diet over time, not to a single food, serving of a recipe or meal.

Choose a diet with plenty of vegetables, fruits and grain products. Vitamins, minerals, fiber and complex carbohydrates abound in these low fat food choices. Filling up on fiber leaves less room for fat and may produce a slight decrease in blood cholesterol levels. Antioxidants such as beta carotene and the vitamins C and E may protect against heart disease, while magnesium, phosphorous and calcium are minerals that may keep blood pressure levels under control.

Use sugars in moderation. The ban on sugar has been lifted for people with diabetes but it is not altogether gone. The new guidelines for simple sugar intake are based on scientific research that indicates that carbohydrate in the form of simple sugars does not raise blood sugar levels more rapidly than any other type of carbohydrate food. What is more important is the total amount of carbohydrate consumed, not the source. However, keep in mind that since simple sugars are loaded with calories, contain no vitamins and minerals, and are linked to the development of cavities, it is still a good idea to limit your intake of simple sugars to no more than 25 percent of total carbohydrate.

Use salt and sodium in moderation. Some people with diabetes may be more sensitive to sodium than others, making them more susceptible to high blood pressure. Minimize this risk by limiting sodium intake to no more than 2,400 mg a day (about 1 teaspoon of salt) and choosing single food items with less than 400 mg of sodium and entrées with less than 800 mg of sodium per serving.

Facts About the Foods

The recipes in this publication were designed for people with diabetes in mind. All are based on the principles of sound nutrition as outlined by the Dietary Guidelines, making them perfect for the entire family. Though the recipes in this publication are not intended as a medically therapeutic program, nor as a substitute for medically approved meal plans for individuals with diabetes, they are low in calories, fat, sodium and cholesterol and will fit easily into an individualized meal plan designed by your physician, registered dietitian and you.

Facts About the Exchanges

The nutrition information that appears with each recipe was calculated by an independent nutrition consulting firm and the Dietary Exchanges are based on the Exchange Lists for Meal Planning developed by American Diabetes Association/The American Dietetic Association. Every effort has been made to check the accuracy of these numbers. However, because numerous variables account for a wide range of values in certain foods, all analyses that appear in this book should be considered approximate.

■ The analysis of each recipe includes all the ingredients that are listed in that recipe, except ingredients labeled as "optional" or "for garnish." Nutritional analysis is provided for the primary recipe only, not for the recipe variations.

■ If a range is offered for an ingredient, the first amount given was used to calculate the nutrition information.

■ If an ingredient is presented with an option ("2 cups hot cooked rice or noodles," for example), the first item listed was used to calculate the nutrition information.

■ Foods shown in photographs on the same serving plate and offered as "serve with" suggestions at the end of a recipe are not included in the recipe analysis unless they are listed in the ingredient list.

■ Meat should be trimmed of all visible fat because this is reflected in the nutritional analysis.

■ In recipes calling for cooked rice or noodles, the analysis was based on rice or noodles that were prepared without added salt and fat.

■ Most processed foods contain a significant amount of sodium and the amount of sodium is reflected in the analysis. Rinsing canned or jarred processed foods such as beans and tuna under cold running water for one minute eliminates between 40 and 60 percent of added sodium.

Appetizers & Snacks

Vegetable-Topped Hummus

Look for tahini, a thick paste made from ground sesame seeds, in Middle Eastern markets, health food stores or the ethnic section of large supermarkets.

    1 can (about 15 ounces) chick-peas, rinsed and drained
    2 tablespoons tahini
    2 tablespoons lemon juice
    1 clove garlic
    ¾ teaspoon salt
    1 tomato, finely chopped
    2 green onions, finely chopped
    2 tablespoons chopped parsley

1. Combine chick-peas, tahini, lemon juice, garlic and salt in food processor; process until smooth.

2. Combine tomato, green onions and parsley in small bowl.

3. Place chick-pea mixture in medium serving bowl; spoon tomato mixture evenly over top. Serve with wedges of pita bread or assorted crackers.

Makes 8 servings

Nutrients per Serving: Calories: 82 (31% Calories from Fat), Total Fat: 3 g, Saturated Fat: trace, Protein: 3 g, Carbohydrate: 11 g, Cholesterol: 0 mg, Sodium: 429 mg, Fiber: 3 g, Sugar: 1 g
Dietary Exchanges: ½ Starch/Bread, 1 Vegetable, ½ Fat

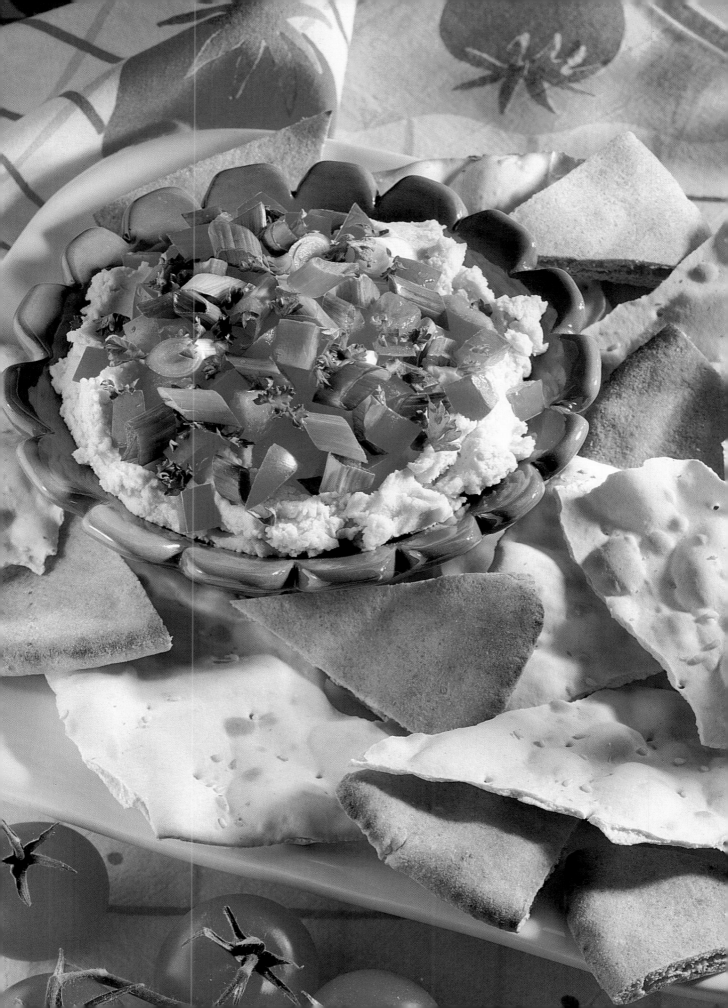

Roasted Eggplant Rolls

2 medium eggplants (¾ pound each)
2 tablespoons lemon juice
1 teaspoon olive oil
4 tablespoons (2 ounces) fat-free cream cheese
2 tablespoons nonfat sour cream
1 green onion, minced
4 sun-dried tomatoes (packed in oil), drained and minced
1 clove garlic, minced
¼ teaspoon dried oregano leaves
⅛ teaspoon black pepper
16 medium spinach leaves, washed, stemmed and dried
1 cup bottled spaghetti sauce

1. Preheat oven to 450°F. Spray 2 nonstick baking sheets with nonstick cooking spray; set aside. Trim ends from eggplants; cut lengthwise into ¼-inch-thick slices. Discard outside slices that are mostly skin. (You will have about 16 slices.)

2. Combine lemon juice and olive oil in small bowl; brush lightly over both sides of eggplant slices. Arrange slices in single layer on baking sheets. Bake 10 to 12 minutes or until slightly golden brown on bottom. Turn slices over and bake 10 to 12 minutes more or until golden on both sides and tender. (Slices may not brown evenly; turn slices as they brown. Some very dark spots will occur.) Transfer slices to plate; cool.

3. Meanwhile, stir cream cheese in small bowl until smooth. Add sour cream, green onion, tomatoes, garlic, oregano and pepper; stir until blended.

4. Place eggplant slices on work surface; spread about 1 teaspoon cream cheese mixture evenly over each slice. Arrange spinach leaves on top leaving ½-inch border. Roll up, beginning at narrower end; lay rolls seam sides down on serving platter. (If making ahead, cover and refrigerate up to 2 days. Bring to room temperature before serving.) Serve with warm spaghetti sauce.   *Makes 8 servings (2 rolls each)*

Nutrients per Serving: Calories: 77 (27% Calories from Fat), Total Fat: 3 g,
Saturated Fat: trace, Protein: 3 g, Carbohydrate: 12 g, Cholesterol: 0 mg,
Sodium: 213 mg, Fiber: trace, Sugar: trace
Dietary Exchanges: 2 Vegetable, ½ Fat

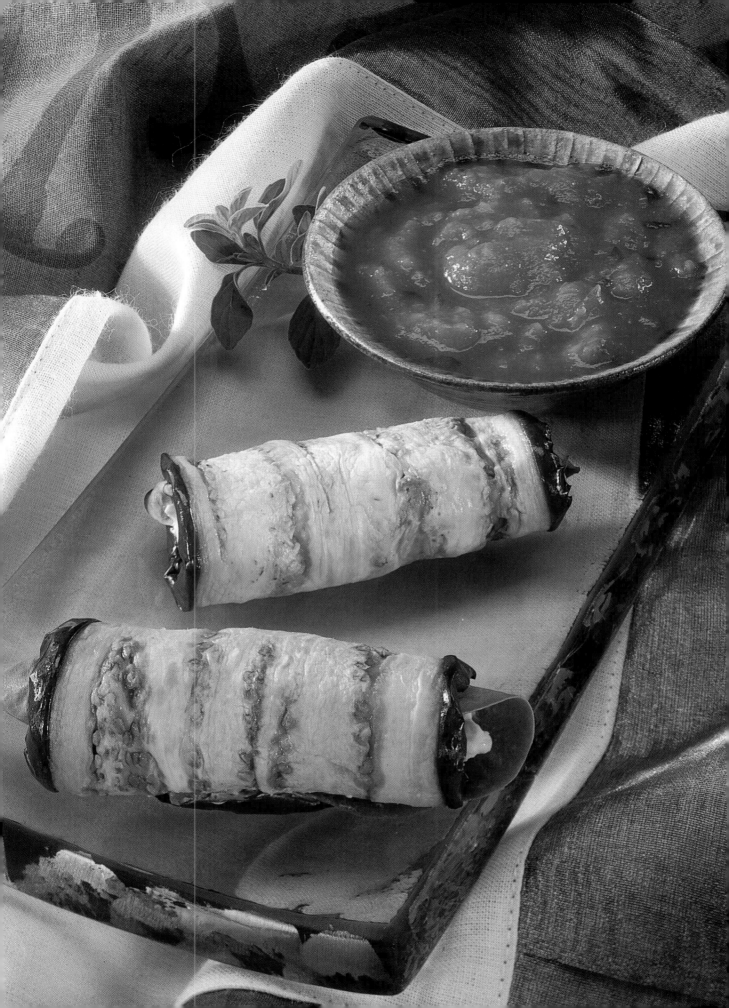

Cinnamon Caramel Corn

8 cups air-popped popcorn (about ⅓ cup kernels)
2 tablespoons honey
4 teaspoons margarine
¼ teaspoon ground cinnamon

1. Preheat oven to 350°F. Spray jelly-roll pan with nonstick cooking spray. Place popcorn in large bowl.

2. Stir honey, margarine and cinnamon in small saucepan over low heat until margarine is melted and mixture is smooth; immediately pour over popcorn. Toss with spoon to coat evenly. Pour onto prepared pan; bake 12 to 14 minutes or until coating is golden brown and appears crackled, stirring twice. Let cool on pan 5 minutes. (As popcorn cools, coating becomes crisp. If not crisp enough, or if popcorn softens upon standing, return to oven and heat 5 to 8 minutes more.)   *Makes 4 servings*

Nutrients per Serving: Calories: 117 (29% Calories from Fat), Total Fat: 4 g, Saturated Fat: 1 g, Protein: 2 g, Carbohydrate: 19 g, Cholesterol: 0 mg, Sodium: 45 mg, Fiber: 1 g, Sugar: 9 g
Dietary Exchanges: 1 Starch/Bread, 1 Fat

Variations

Cajun Popcorn: Preheat oven and prepare jelly-roll pan as directed above. Combine 7 teaspoons honey, 4 teaspoons margarine and 1 teaspoon Cajun or Creole seasoning in small saucepan. Proceed with recipe as directed above. Makes 4 servings.

Nutrients per Serving: Calories: 122 (28% Calories from Fat), Total Fat: 4 g, Saturated Fat: 1 g, Protein: 2 g, Carbohydrate: 20 g, Cholesterol: 0 mg, Sodium: 91 mg, Fiber: 1 g, Sugar: 10 g
Dietary Exchanges: 1½ Starch/Bread, ½ Fat

Italian Popcorn: Spray 8 cups of air-popped popcorn with fat-free butter-flavored spray to coat. Sprinkle with 2 tablespoons finely grated Parmesan cheese, ⅛ teaspoon black pepper and ½ teaspoon dried oregano leaves. Gently toss to coat. Makes 4 servings.

Nutrients per Serving: Calories: 65 (14% Calories from Fat), Total Fat: 1 g, Saturated Fat: 1 g, Protein: 3 g, Carbohydrate: 10 g, Cholesterol: 2 mg, Sodium: 58 mg, Fiber: 1 g, Sugar: 0 g
Dietary Exchanges: 1 Starch/Bread

Clockwise from top: Italian Popcorn,
Cinnamon Caramel Corn
and Cajun Popcorn

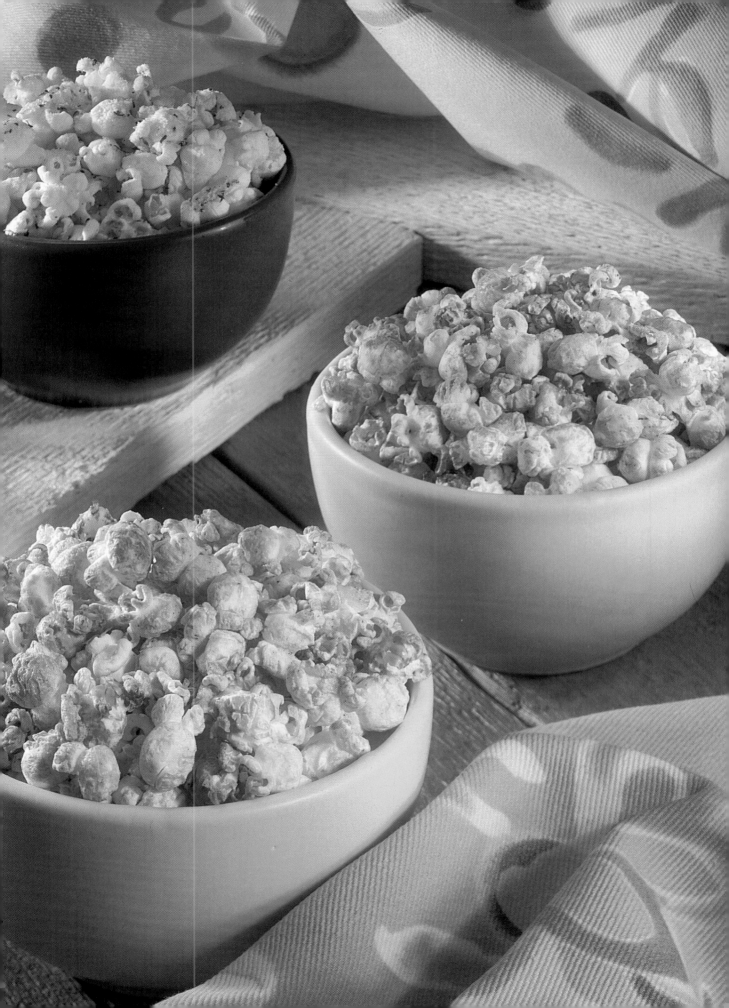

Greek Spinach-Cheese Rolls

Keep these savory rolls on hand for a quick pick-me-up or serve along side soup or salad.

1 loaf (1 pound) frozen bread dough
1 package (10 ounces) frozen chopped spinach, thawed and
** squeezed dry**
¾ cup (3 ounces) crumbled feta cheese
½ cup (2 ounces) shredded reduced-fat Monterey Jack cheese
4 green onions, thinly sliced
1 teaspoon dried dill weed
½ teaspoon garlic powder
½ teaspoon black pepper

1. Thaw bread dough according to package directions. Spray 15 muffin cups with nonstick cooking spray; set aside. Roll out dough on lightly floured surface to 15×9-inch rectangle. (If dough is springy and difficult to roll, cover with plastic wrap and let rest 5 minutes to relax.) Position dough so long edge runs parallel to edge of work surface.

2. Combine spinach, cheeses, green onions, dill weed, garlic powder and pepper in large bowl; mix well.

3. Sprinkle spinach mixture evenly over dough to within 1 inch of long edges. Starting at long edge, roll up snugly, pinching seam closed. Place seam side down; cut roll with serrated knife into 1-inch-wide slices. Place slices cut sides up in prepared muffin cups. Cover with plastic wrap; let stand 30 minutes in warm place until rolls are slightly puffy.

4. Preheat oven to 375°F. Bake 20 to 25 minutes or until golden. Serve warm or at room temperature. Rolls can be stored in refrigerator in airtight container up to 2 days.   *Makes 15 servings (1 roll each)*

Nutrients per Serving: Calories: 111 (24% Calories from Fat), Total Fat: 3 g,
Saturated Fat: 2 g, Protein: 5 g, Carbohydrate: 16 g, Cholesterol: 8 mg,
Sodium: 267 mg, Fiber: trace, Sugar: trace
Dietary Exchanges: 1 Starch/Bread, ½ Lean Meat, ½ Fat

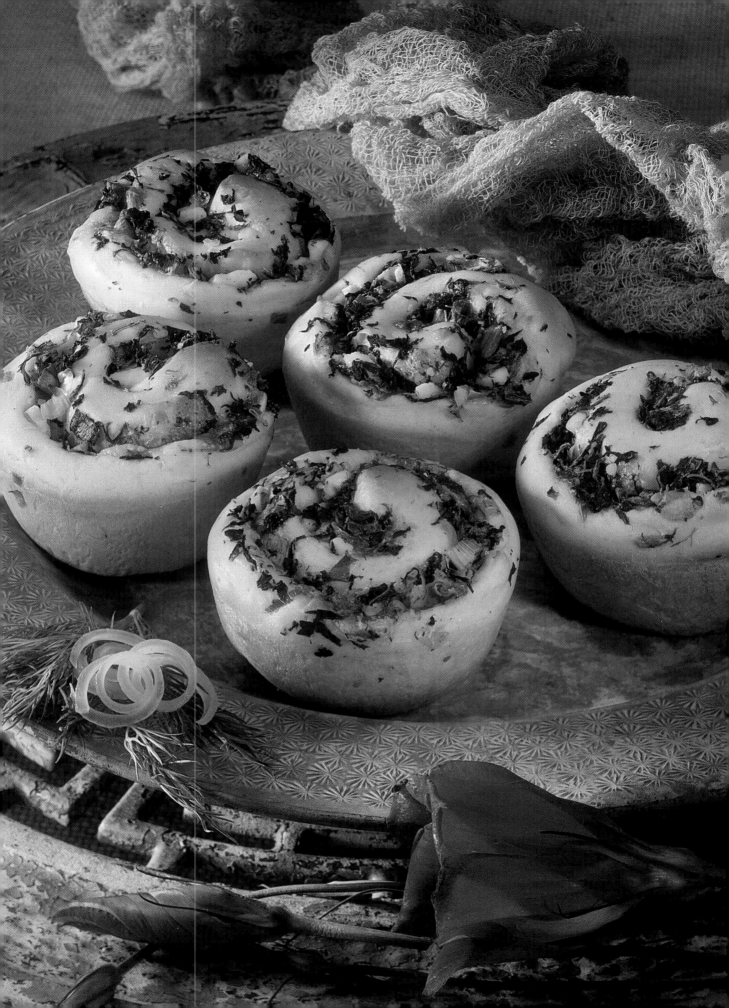

Venezuelan Salsa

Try a taste-tempting tropical sensation! This unusual salsa makes a terrific appetizer, or serve it with fruit salads, grilled chicken or fish.

  1 mango, peeled, pitted and diced
½ medium papaya, peeled, seeded and diced
½ medium avocado, peeled, pitted and diced
  1 carrot, finely chopped
  1 small onion, finely chopped
  1 rib celery, finely chopped
    Juice of 1 lemon
  3 cloves garlic, minced
  2 tablespoons chopped cilantro
  1 jalapeño pepper,* finely chopped
1½ teaspoons ground cumin
½ teaspoon salt

*Jalapeño peppers can sting and irritate the skin; wear rubber gloves when handling peppers and do not touch eyes. Wash hands after handling.

1. Combine all ingredients in medium bowl. Refrigerate several hours to allow flavors to blend. Serve with baked tortilla chips, carrot and celery sticks or apple wedges.   *Makes 10 servings (¼ cup each)*

Nutrients per Serving: Calories: 52 (27% Calories from Fat), Total Fat: 2 g, Saturated Fat: trace, Protein: 1 g, Carbohydrate: 9 g, Cholesterol: 0 mg, Sodium: 117 mg, Fiber: 2 g, Sugar: 5 g
Dietary Exchanges: 1 Fruit

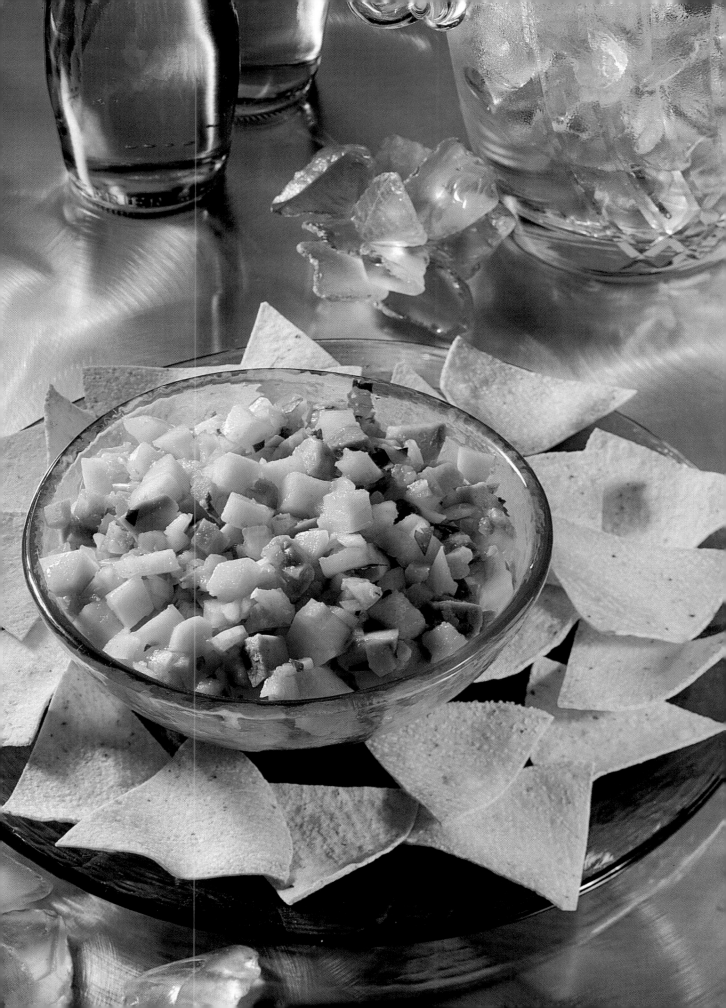

Banana & Chocolate Chip Pops

Three-ounce paper cups can be used in place of popsicle molds. Spoon yogurt mixture into paper cups, insert wooden stick in center of each and freeze. To prevent popsicles from tipping over, simply stand cups in a muffin pan after filling. To unmold, peel paper cup away.

1 small ripe banana
1 carton (8 ounces) banana nonfat yogurt
⅛ teaspoon ground nutmeg
2 tablespoons mini chocolate chips

1. Slice banana; place in food processor with yogurt and nutmeg. Process until smooth. Transfer to small bowl; stir in chips.

2. Spoon banana mixture into 4 plastic popsicle molds. Place tops on molds; set in provided stand. Set on level surface in freezer; freeze 2 hours or until firm. To unmold, briefly run warm water over popsicle molds until each pop loosens.   *Makes 4 servings*

Nutrients per Serving: Calories: 103 (14% Calories from Fat), Total Fat: 2 g, Saturated Fat: trace, Protein: 3 g, Carbohydrate: 20 g, Cholesterol: 1 mg, Sodium: 37 mg, Fiber: trace, Sugar: 16 g
Dietary Exchanges: 1½ Fruit

Variations

Peanut Butter & Jelly Pops: Stir ¼ cup reduced-fat peanut butter in small bowl until smooth; stir in 1 carton (8 ounces) vanilla nonfat yogurt. Drop 2 tablespoons all-fruit strawberry preserves on top of mixture; pull spoon back and forth through mixture several times to swirl slightly. Spoon into 4 molds and freeze as directed above. Makes 4 servings.

Nutrients per Serving: Calories: 169 (32% Calories from Fat), Total Fat: 6 g, Saturated Fat: 1 g, Protein: 7 g, Carbohydrate: 21 g, Cholesterol: 0 mg, Sodium: 131 mg, Fiber: 1 g, Sugar: 1 g
Dietary Exchanges: 1½ Starch/Bread, ½ Lean Meat, 1 Fat

Blueberry-Lime Pops: Stir 1 carton (8 ounces) Key lime nonfat yogurt in small bowl until smooth; fold in ⅓ cup frozen blueberries. Spoon into 4 molds and freeze as directed above. Makes 4 servings.

Nutrients per Serving: Calories: 57 (1% Calories from Fat), Total Fat: trace, Saturated Fat: trace, Protein: 2 g, Carbohydrate: 12 g, Cholesterol: 0 mg, Sodium: 32 mg, Fiber: trace, Sugar: 10 g
Dietary Exchanges: 1 Fruit

Clockwise from top: Peanut Butter & Jelly Pop, Blueberry-Lime Pop and Banana & Chocolate Chip Pop

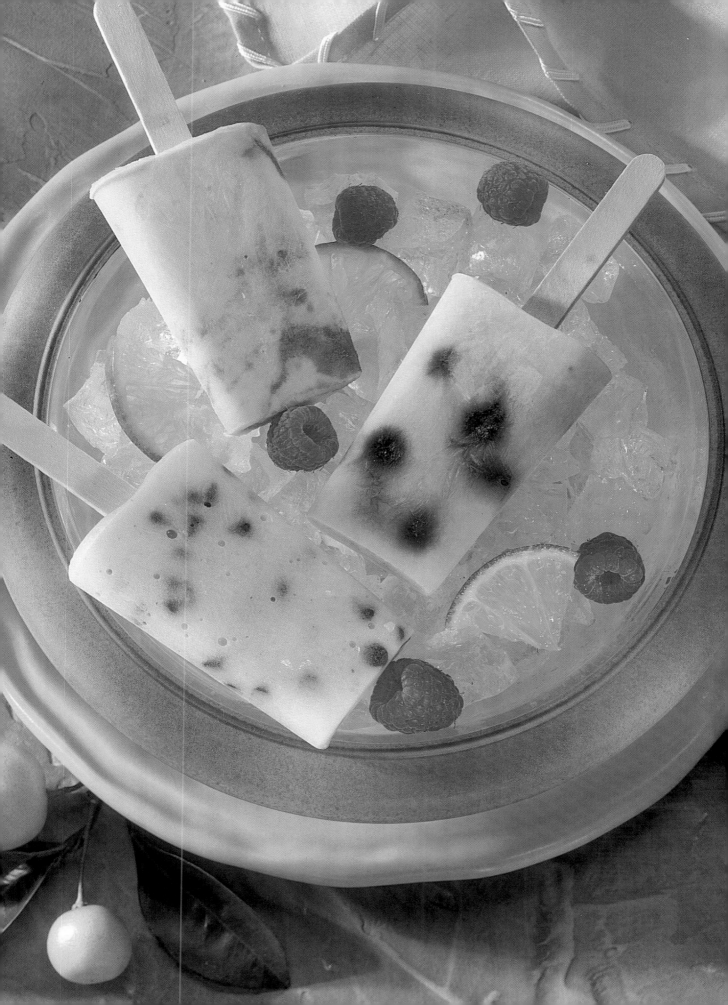

Tuscan White Bean Crostini

For a refreshing light lunch, serve the white bean mixture as a salad on a bed of Bibb lettuce leaves.

2 cans (15 ounces each) white beans (such as Great Northern or cannellini), rinsed and drained
½ large red bell pepper, finely chopped *or* ⅓ cup finely chopped roasted red bell pepper
⅓ cup finely chopped onion
⅓ cup red wine vinegar
3 tablespoons chopped parsley
1 tablespoon olive oil
2 cloves garlic, minced
½ teaspoon dried oregano leaves
¼ teaspoon black pepper
18 French bread slices, about ¼ inch thick

1. Combine beans, bell pepper and onion in large bowl.

2. Whisk together vinegar, parsley, oil, garlic, oregano and black pepper in small bowl. Pour over bean mixture; toss to coat. Cover; refrigerate 2 hours or overnight.

3. Arrange bread slices in single layer on large nonstick baking sheet or broiler pan. Broil, 6 to 8 inches from heat, 30 to 45 seconds or until bread slices are lightly toasted. Remove; cool completely.

4. Top each toasted bread slice with about 3 tablespoons of bean mixture.

Makes 6 servings

Nutrients per Serving: Calories: 317 (12% Calories from Fat), Total Fat: 4 g,
Saturated Fat: 1 g, Protein: 15 g, Carbohydrate: 57 g, Cholesterol: 0 mg,
Sodium: 800 mg, Fiber: 1 g, Sugar: trace
Dietary Exchanges: 2 Starch/Bread, 1 Vegetable, ½ Fat

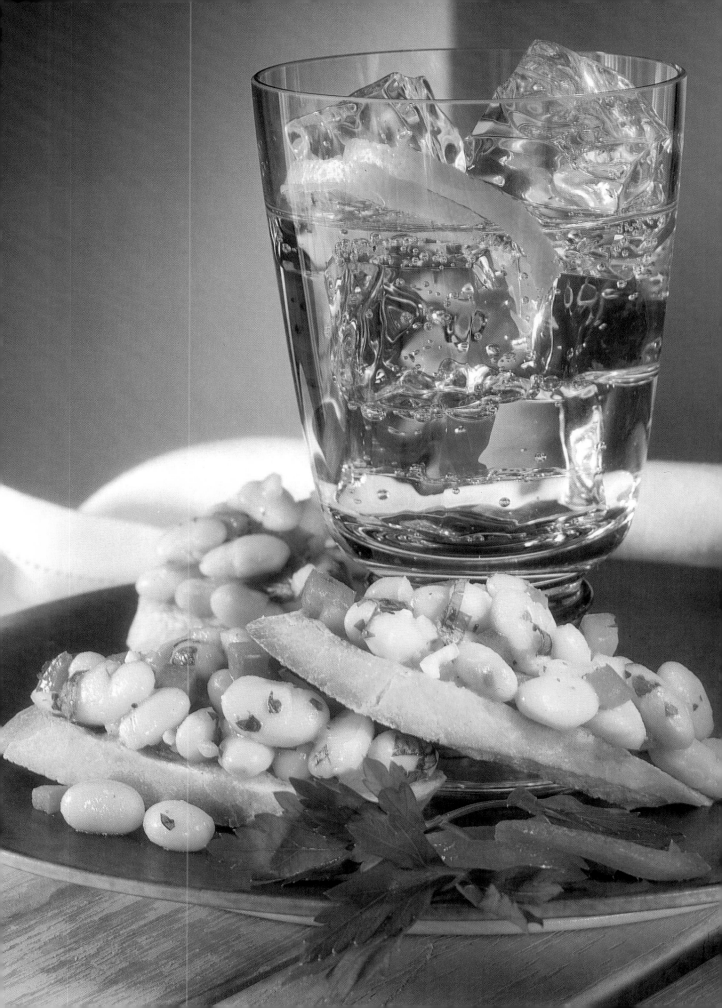

Apricot-Chicken Pot Stickers

2 cups plus 1 tablespoon water, divided
2 small boneless skinless chicken breasts (about 8 ounces)
2 cups chopped finely shredded cabbage
½ cup all-fruit apricot preserves
2 green onions with tops, finely chopped
2 teaspoons soy sauce
½ teaspoon grated fresh ginger
⅛ teaspoon black pepper
30 (3-inch) wonton wrappers
   Prepared sweet & sour sauce (optional)

1. Bring 2 cups water to boil in medium saucepan. Add chicken. Reduce heat to low; simmer, covered, 10 minutes or until chicken is no longer pink in center. Remove from saucepan; drain.

2. Add cabbage and remaining 1 tablespoon water to saucepan. Cook over high heat 1 to 2 minutes or until water evaporates, stirring occasionally. Remove from heat; cool slightly.

3. Finely chop chicken. Add to saucepan along with preserves, green onions, soy sauce, ginger and pepper; mix well.

4. To assemble pot stickers, remove 3 wonton wrappers at a time from package. Spoon slightly rounded tablespoonful of chicken mixture onto center of each wrapper; brush edges with water. Bring 4 corners together; press to seal. Repeat with remaining wrappers and filling.

5. Spray steamer with nonstick cooking spray. Assemble steamer so that water is ½ inch below steamer basket. Fill steamer basket with pot stickers, leaving enough space between them to prevent sticking. Cover; steam 5 minutes. Transfer pot stickers to serving plate. Serve with prepared sweet & sour sauce, if desired.   *Makes 10 servings (3 pot stickers each)*

Nutrients per Serving: Calories: 145 (6% Calories from Fat), Total Fat: 1 g,
Saturated Fat: trace, Protein: 8 g, Carbohydrate: 26 g, Cholesterol: 17 mg,
Sodium: 223 mg, Fiber: 1 g, Sugar: 10 g
Dietary Exchanges: 1½ Starch/Bread, ½ Lean Meat

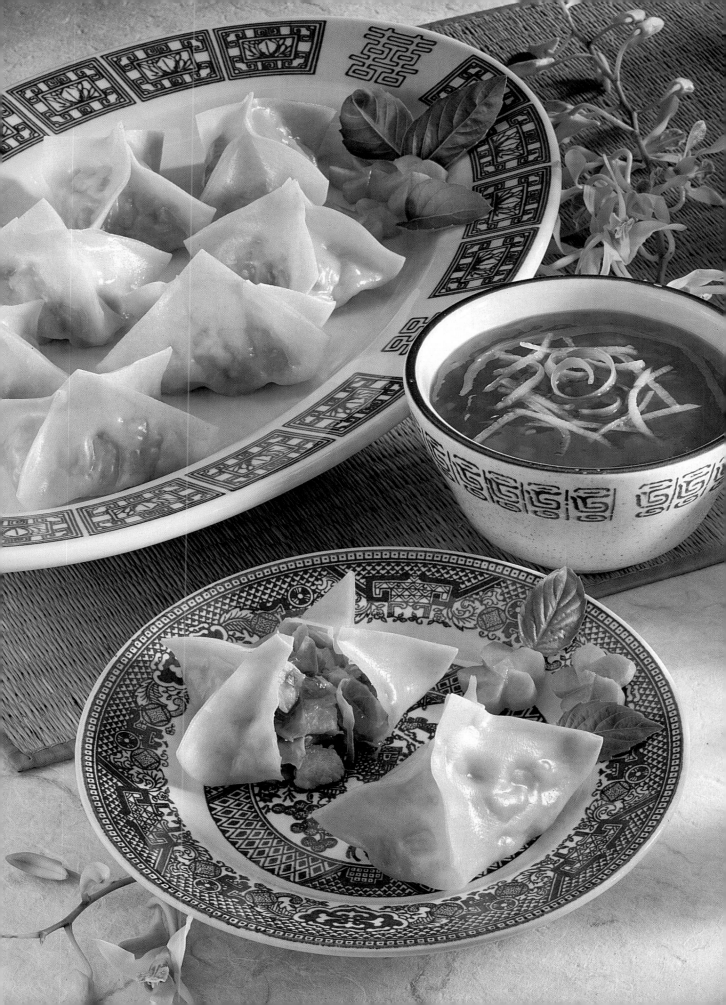

Soups & Salads

Italian Crouton Salad

   6 ounces French or Italian bread
   ¼ cup plain nonfat yogurt
   ¼ cup red wine vinegar
   4 teaspoons olive oil
   1 tablespoon water
   3 cloves garlic, minced
   6 medium (about 12 ounces) plum tomatoes
   ½ medium red onion, thinly sliced
   3 tablespoons slivered fresh basil leaves
   2 tablespoons finely chopped parsley
   12 leaves red leaf lettuce *or* 4 cups prepared Italian salad mix
   2 tablespoons grated Parmesan cheese

1. Preheat broiler. Cut bread into ¾-inch cubes. Place in single layer on jelly-roll pan. Broil, 4 inches from heat, 3 minutes or until bread is golden, stirring every 30 seconds to 1 minute. Remove from baking sheet; place in large bowl.

2. Whisk together yogurt, vinegar, oil, water and garlic in small bowl until blended; set aside. Core tomatoes; cut into ¼-inch-wide slices. Add to bread along with onion, basil and parsley; stir until blended. Pour yogurt mixture over crouton mixture; toss to coat. Cover; refrigerate 30 minutes or up to 1 day. (Croutons will be more tender the following day.)

3. To serve, place lettuce on plates. Spoon crouton mixture over lettuce. Sprinkle with Parmesan cheese. *Makes 6 servings*

Nutrients per Serving: Calories: 160 (28% Calories from Fat), Total Fat: 5 g, Saturated Fat: 1 g, Protein: 6 g, Carbohydrate: 25 g, Cholesterol: 2 mg, Sodium: 234 mg, Fiber: 2 g, Sugar: 5 g
Dietary Exchanges: 1 Starch/Bread, 1½ Vegetable, 1 Fat

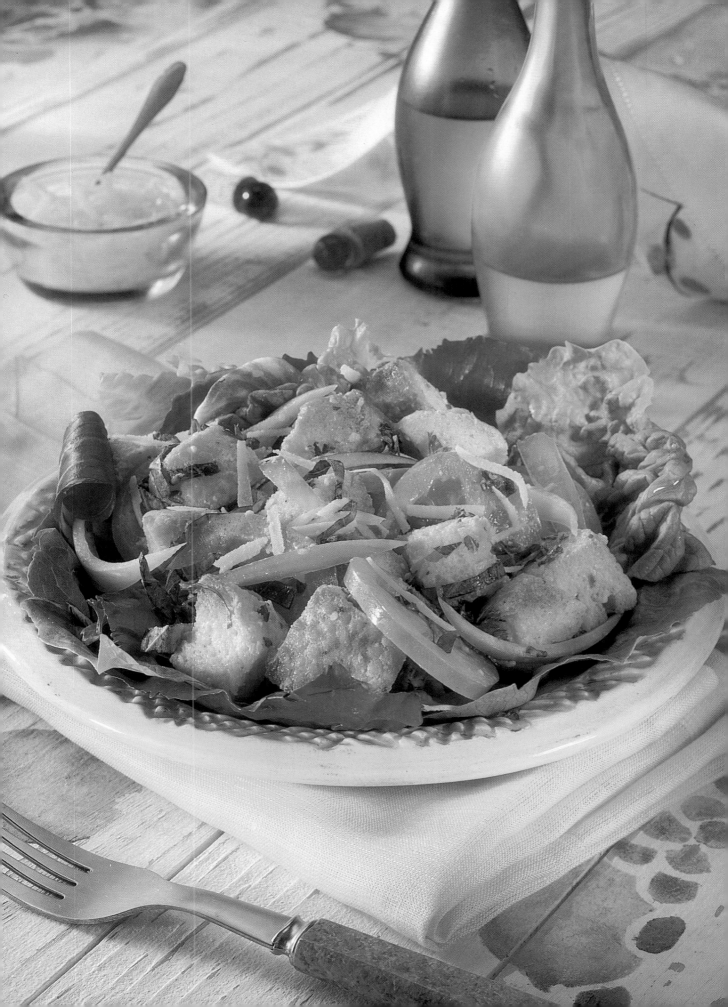

Indian Carrot Soup

Vitamin-rich and inexpensive, carrots star in this rich and spicy soup without the addition of any cream. This soup can be made with winter squash, such as butternut, acorn or hubbard, in place of the carrots.

Nonstick cooking spray
1 small onion, chopped
1 tablespoon minced fresh ginger
1 teaspoon olive oil
1½ teaspoons curry powder
½ teaspoon ground cumin
2 cans (about 14 ounces each) fat-free reduced-sodium chicken broth, divided
1 pound peeled baby carrots
1 tablespoon sugar
¼ teaspoon ground cinnamon
Pinch ground red pepper
2 teaspoons fresh lime juice
3 tablespoons chopped cilantro
¼ cup plain nonfat yogurt

1. Spray large saucepan with cooking spray; heat over medium heat. Add onion and ginger; reduce heat to low. Cover; cook 3 to 4 minutes or until onion is transparent and crisp-tender, stirring occasionally. Add olive oil; cook and stir, uncovered, 3 to 4 minutes or until onion just turns golden. Add curry powder and cumin; cook and stir 30 seconds or until fragrant. Add 1 can chicken broth and carrots; bring to a boil over high heat. Reduce heat to low; simmer, covered, 15 minutes or until carrots are tender.

2. Ladle carrot mixture into food processor; process until smooth. Return to saucepan; stir in remaining 1 can chicken broth, sugar, cinnamon and red pepper; bring to a boil over medium heat. Remove from heat; stir in lime juice. Ladle into bowls; sprinkle with cilantro. Top each serving with 1 tablespoon yogurt.   *Makes 4 servings*

Nutrients per Serving: Calories: 99 (20% Calories from Fat), Total Fat: 2 g, Saturated Fat: trace, Protein: 3 g, Carbohydrate: 17 g, Cholesterol: trace, Sodium: 77 mg, Fiber: 1 g, Sugar: 4 g
Dietary Exchanges: ½ Starch/Bread, 3 Vegetable, 1 Fat

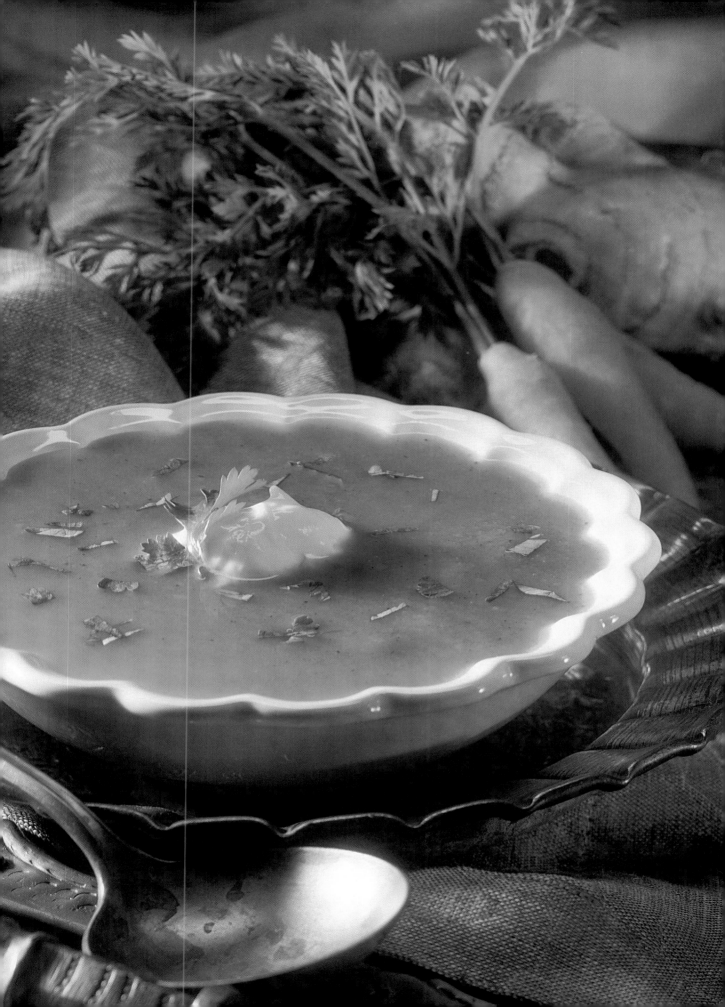

Caribbean Cole Slaw

Mangoes add a tropical twist to this familiar salad and provide plenty of vitamins A and C.

Orange-Mango Dressing (recipe follows)
8 cups shredded green cabbage
1½ large mangoes, peeled, pitted and diced
½ medium red bell pepper, thinly sliced
½ medium yellow bell pepper, thinly sliced
6 green onions, thinly sliced
¼ cup chopped cilantro

1. Prepare Orange-Mango Dressing.

2. Combine cabbage, mangoes, bell peppers, green onions and cilantro in large bowl; stir gently to mix evenly. Pour in Orange-Mango Dressing; toss gently to coat. Serve, or store in refrigerator up to 1 day.

Makes 6 servings

Orange-Mango Dressing

½ mango, peeled, pitted and cubed
1 carton (6 ounces) plain nonfat yogurt
¼ cup frozen orange juice concentrate
3 tablespoons fresh lime juice
½ to 1 jalapeño pepper,* stemmed, seeded and minced
1 teaspoon finely minced fresh ginger

*Jalapeño peppers can sting and irritate the skin; wear rubber gloves when handling peppers and do not touch eyes. Wash hands after handling.

1. Place mango in food processor; process until smooth. Add remaining ingredients; process until smooth.

Makes about 1 cup

Nutrients per Serving: Calories: 124 (4% Calories from Fat), Total Fat: 1 g, Saturated Fat: trace, Protein: 4 g, Carbohydrate: 28 g, Cholesterol: 1 mg, Sodium: 52 mg, Fiber: 4 g, Sugar: 16 g
Dietary Exchanges: 2 Fruit

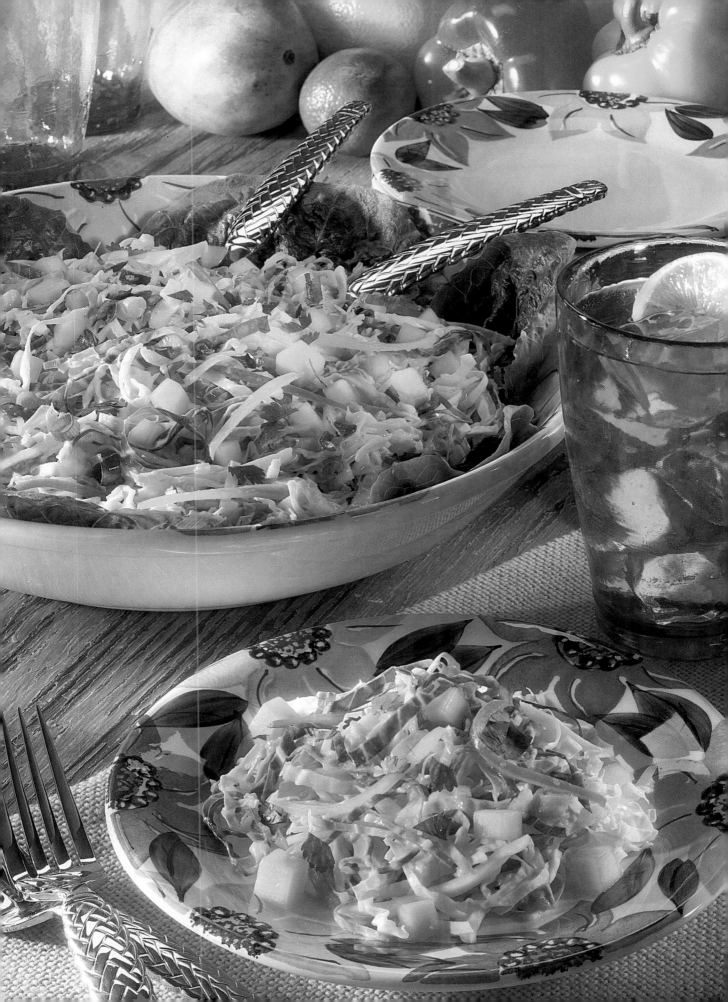

Southwest Corn and Turkey Soup

Dry chilies add a rich earthy flavor not achievable with their fresh counterparts.

3 dried ancho chilies (each about 4 inches long) *or* **6 dried New
    Mexico chilies (each about 6 inches long)**
2 small zucchini
    Nonstick cooking spray
1 medium onion, thinly sliced
3 cloves garlic, minced
1 teaspoon ground cumin
3 cans (about 14 ounces each) fat-free reduced-sodium chicken broth
1½ to 2 cups (8 to 12 ounces) shredded cooked dark turkey meat
1 can (15 ounces) chick-peas or black beans, rinsed and drained
1 package (10 ounces) frozen corn
¼ cup cornmeal
1 teaspoon dried oregano leaves
⅓ cup chopped cilantro

1. Cut stems from chilies; shake out seeds. Place chilies in medium bowl; cover with boiling water. Let stand 20 to 40 minutes or until chilies are soft; drain. Cut open lengthwise and lay flat on work surface. With edge of small knife, scrape chili pulp from skin (thicker-skinned ancho chilies will yield more flesh than thinner-skinned New Mexico chilies). Finely mince pulp; set aside.

2. Cut zucchini in half lengthwise; slice crosswise into ½-inch-wide pieces. Set aside.

3. Spray large saucepan with cooking spray; heat over medium heat. Add onion; cook, covered, 3 to 4 minutes or until light golden brown, stirring several times. Add garlic and cumin; cook and stir about 30 seconds or until fragrant. Add chicken broth, reserved chili pulp, zucchini, turkey, chick-peas, corn, cornmeal and oregano; bring to a boil over high heat. Reduce heat to low; simmer 15 minutes or until zucchini is tender. Stir in cilantro; ladle into bowls and serve.   *Makes 6 servings*

Nutrients per Serving: Calories: 243 (19% Calories from Fat), Total Fat: 5 g,
Saturated Fat: 1 g, Protein: 19 g, Carbohydrate: 32 g, Cholesterol: 32 mg,
Sodium: 408 mg, Fiber: 7 g, Sugar: 2 g
Dietary Exchanges: 2 Bread/Starch, 2 Lean Meat

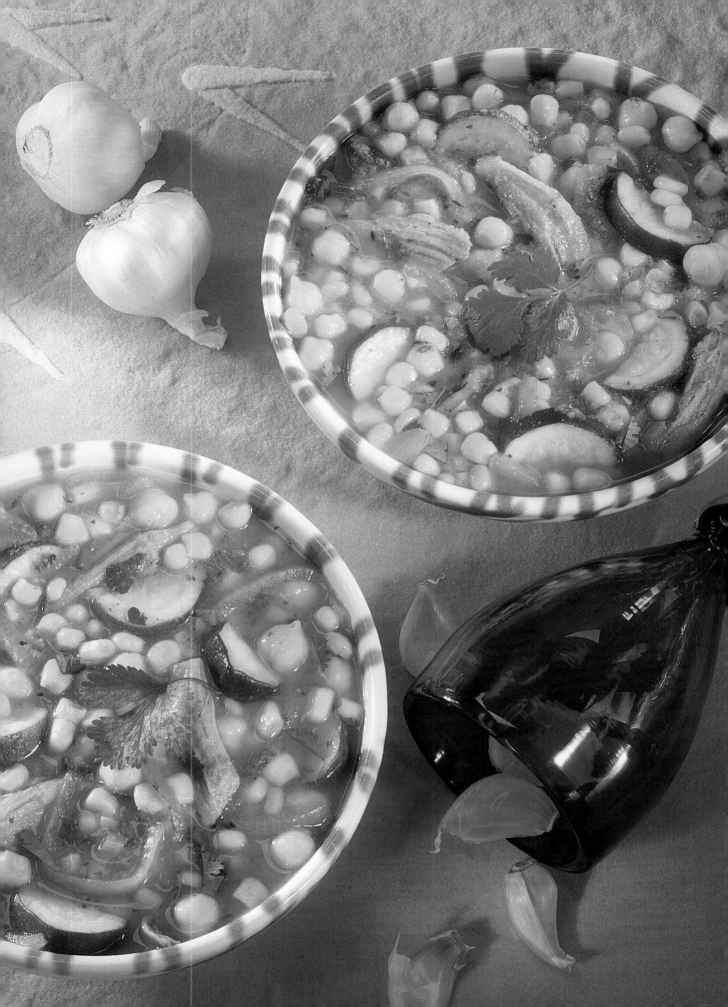

Scallop and Spinach Salad

The combination of scallops, blue cheese and toasted walnuts turn the familiar spinach salad into a delicious new creation.

> **1 package (10 ounces) spinach leaves, washed, stemmed and torn**
> **3 thin slices red onion, halved and separated**
> **12 ounces sea scallops**
> **Ground red pepper**
> **Paprika**
> **Nonstick cooking spray**
> **½ cup prepared fat-free Italian salad dressing**
> **¼ cup crumbled blue cheese**
> **2 tablespoons toasted walnuts**

1. Pat spinach dry; place in large bowl with red onion. Cover; set aside.

2. Rinse scallops. Cut in half horizontally (to make 2 thin rounds); pat dry. Sprinkle top side lightly with red pepper and paprika. Spray large nonstick skillet with cooking spray; heat over high heat until very hot. Add half of scallops, seasoned side down, in single layer, placing ½ inch or more apart. Sprinkle with red pepper and paprika. Cook 2 minutes or until browned on bottom. Turn scallops; cook 1 to 2 minutes or until opaque in center. Transfer to plate; cover to keep warm. Wipe skillet clean; repeat procedure with remaining scallops.

3. Place dressing in small saucepan; bring to a boil over high heat. Pour dressing over spinach and onion; toss to coat. Divide among 4 plates. Place scallops on top of spinach; sprinkle with blue cheese and walnuts.

Makes 4 servings

Nutrients per Serving: Calories: 169 (29% Calories from Fat), Total Fat: 6 g, Saturated Fat: 2 g, Protein: 24 g, Carbohydrate: 6 g, Cholesterol: 50 mg, Sodium: 660 mg, Fiber: 2 g, Sugar: trace
Dietary Exchanges: 3 Lean Meat, 1 Vegetable

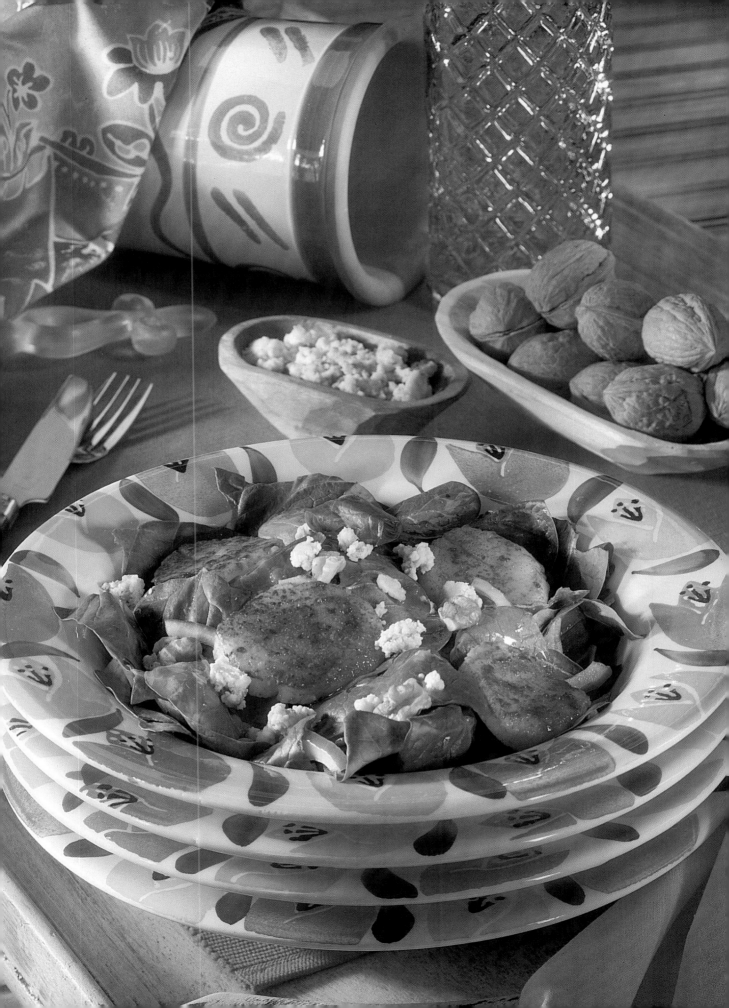

Vietnamese Beef Soup

¾ **pound boneless lean beef, such as sirloin or round steak**
3 **cups water**
1 **can (about 14 ounces) beef broth**
1 **can (10½ ounces) condensed consommé**
2 **tablespoons reduced-sodium soy sauce**
2 **tablespoons minced fresh ginger**
1 **cinnamon stick (3 inches long)**
4 **ounces rice noodles (rice sticks), about ⅛ inch wide**
½ **cup thinly sliced or julienned carrots**
2 **cups fresh mung bean sprouts**
1 **small red onion, halved and thinly sliced**
½ **cup chopped cilantro**
½ **cup chopped fresh basil leaves**
2 **jalapeño peppers,* stemmed, seeded and minced** *or* **1 to
    3 teaspoons Chinese chili sauce or paste**

*Jalapeño peppers can sting and irritate the skin; wear rubber gloves when handling
peppers and do not touch eyes. Wash hands after handling.

1. Place beef in freezer 45 minutes or until firm. Meanwhile, combine
water, beef broth, consommé, soy sauce, ginger and cinnamon stick in
large saucepan; bring to a boil over high heat. Reduce heat to low; simmer, covered, 20 to 30 minutes. Remove cinnamon stick; discard. Meanwhile, place rice noodles in large bowl and cover with warm water; let
stand until pliable, about 20 minutes.

2. Slice beef across grain into very thin strips. Drain noodles. Place
noodles and carrots in simmering broth; cook 2 to 3 minutes or until
noodles are tender. Add beef and bean sprouts; cook 1 minute or until
beef is no longer pink.

3. Remove from heat; stir in red onion, cilantro, basil and jalapeño
peppers. To serve, lift noodles from soup with fork and place in bowls.
Ladle remaining ingredients and broth over noodles.   *Makes 6 servings*

Nutrients per Serving: Calories: 180 (15% Calories from Fat), Total Fat: 3 g,
Saturated Fat: 1 g, Protein: 16 g, Carbohydrate: 23 g, Cholesterol: 32 mg,
Sodium: 800 mg, Fiber: 1 g, Sugar: 3 g
Dietary Exchanges: 1 Starch/Bread, 1½ Lean Meat, 1 Vegetable

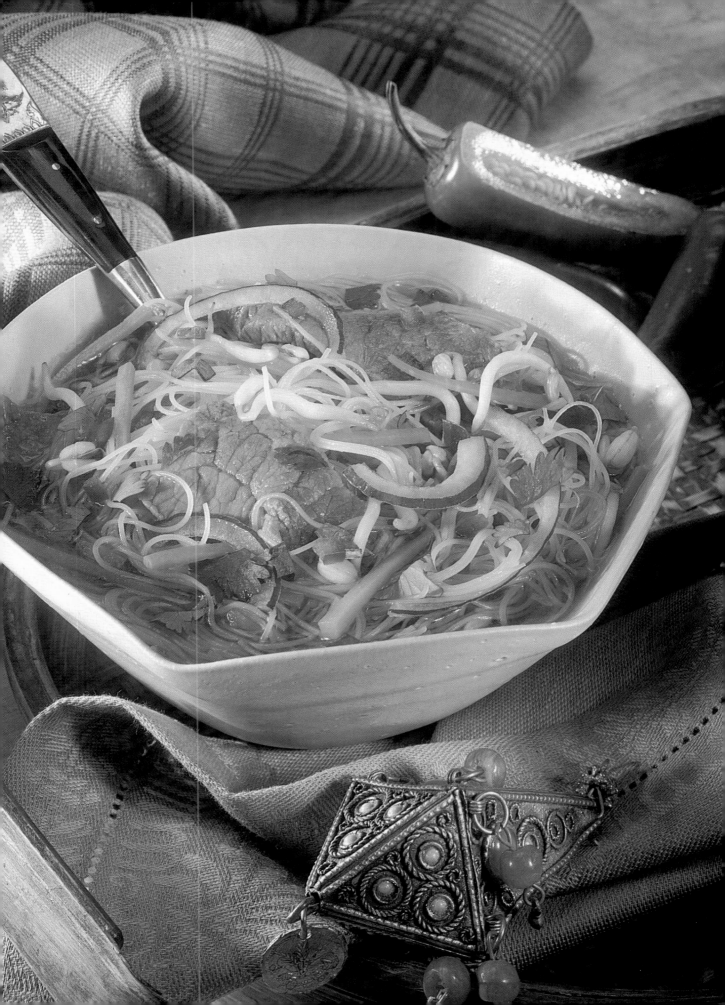

Moroccan Lentil & Vegetable Soup

Not only do lentils taste good, but they are also high in soluble fiber, which lowers blood cholesterol.

   1 tablespoon olive oil
   1 cup chopped onion
   4 medium cloves garlic, minced
  ½ cup dry lentils, sorted, rinsed and drained
 1½ teaspoons ground coriander
 1½ teaspoons ground cumin
  ½ teaspoon black pepper
  ½ teaspoon ground cinnamon
3¾ cups fat-free reduced-sodium chicken broth
  ½ cup chopped celery
  ½ cup chopped sun-dried tomatoes (not packed in oil)
  1 medium yellow summer squash, chopped
  ½ cup chopped green bell pepper
  ½ cup chopped parsley
  1 cup chopped plum tomatoes
  ¼ cup chopped cilantro or basil

1. Heat oil in medium saucepan over medium heat. Add onion and garlic; cook 4 to 5 minutes or until onion is tender, stirring occasionally. Stir in lentils, coriander, cumin, black pepper and cinnamon; cook 2 minutes. Add chicken broth, celery and sun-dried tomatoes; bring to a boil over high heat. Reduce heat to low; simmer, covered, 25 minutes.

2. Stir in squash, bell pepper and parsley. Continue cooking, covered, 10 minutes or until lentils are tender.

3. Top with plum tomatoes and cilantro just before serving.

Makes 6 servings

Nutrients per Serving: Calories: 131 (20% Calories from Fat), Total Fat: 3 g,
Saturated Fat: trace, Protein: 8 g, Carbohydrate: 20 g, Cholesterol: 0 mg,
Sodium: 264 mg, Fiber: 2 g, Sugar: 2 g
Dietary Exchanges: 1 Starch/Bread, 1 Vegetable, ½ Fat

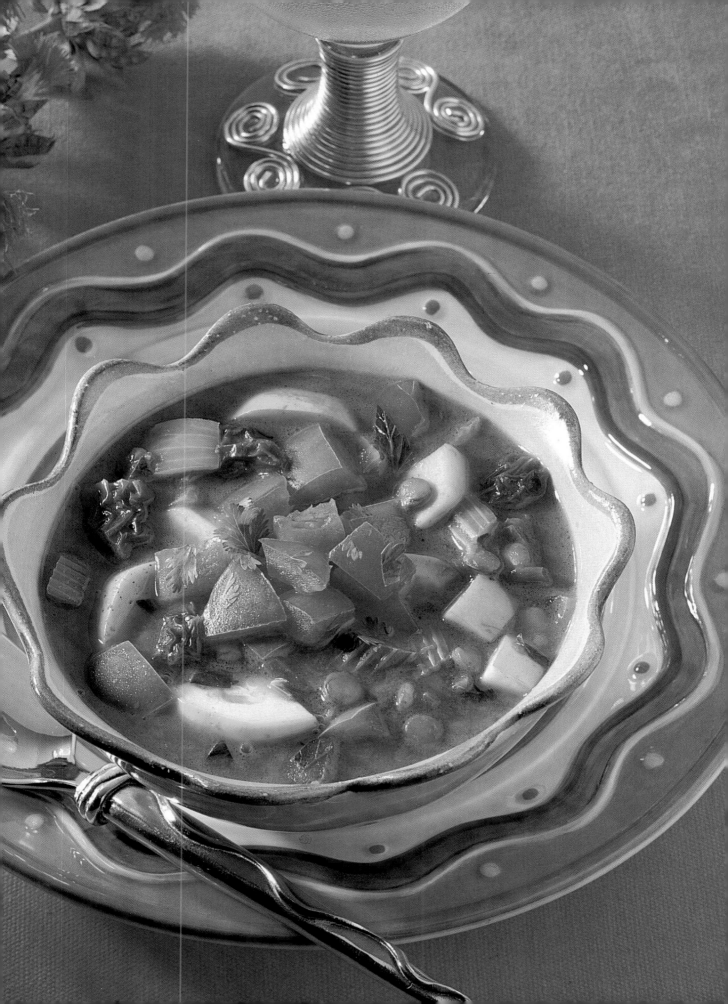

Side Dishes

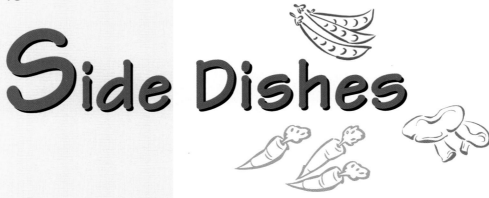

Spicy Chick-Peas & Couscous

Couscous is a grain-like semolina pasta used in northern African cuisines.

> 1 can (about 14 ounces) vegetable broth
> 1 teaspoon ground coriander
> ½ teaspoon ground cardamom
> ½ teaspoon turmeric
> ½ teaspoon hot pepper sauce
> ¼ teaspoon salt
> ⅛ teaspoon cinnamon
> 1 cup julienned carrots
> 1 can (15 ounces) chick-peas, rinsed and drained
> 1 cup frozen peas
> 1 cup quick-cooking couscous
> 2 tablespoons chopped fresh mint or parsley

1. Combine vegetable broth, coriander, cardamom, turmeric, pepper sauce, salt and cinnamon in large saucepan; bring to a boil over high heat. Add carrots; reduce heat and simmer 5 minutes. Add chick-peas and peas; return to a simmer. Simmer, uncovered, 2 minutes.

2. Stir in couscous. Cover; remove from heat. Let stand 5 minutes or until liquid is absorbed. Sprinkle with mint.   *Makes 6 servings*

Nutrients per Serving: Calories: 226 (6% Calories from Fat), Total Fat: 2 g,
Saturated Fat: trace, Protein: 9 g, Carbohydrate: 44 g, Cholesterol: 0 mg,
Sodium: 431 mg, Fiber: 10 g, Sugar: 3 g
Dietary Exchanges: 3 Starch/Bread

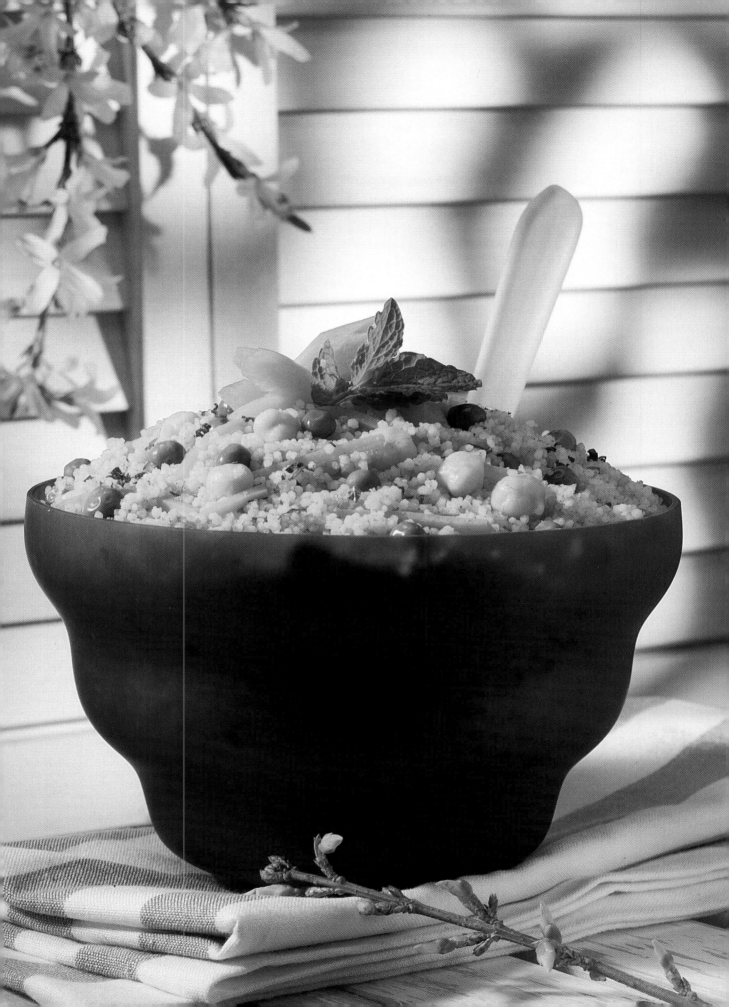

Zucchini Shanghai Style

   4 dried Chinese black mushrooms
   ½ cup fat-free reduced-sodium chicken broth
   2 tablespoons ketchup
   2 teaspoons dry sherry
   1 teaspoon low-sodium soy sauce
   1 teaspoon red wine vinegar
   ¼ teaspoon sugar
 1½ teaspoons vegetable oil, divided
   1 teaspoon minced fresh ginger
   1 clove garlic, minced
   1 large tomato, peeled, seeded and chopped
   1 green onion, finely chopped
   4 tablespoons water, divided
   1 teaspoon cornstarch
   1 pound zucchini (about 3 medium), diagonally cut into 1-inch pieces
   ½ small yellow onion, cut into wedges and separated

1. Soak mushrooms in warm water 20 minutes. Drain, reserving ¼ cup liquid. Squeeze out excess water. Discard stems; slice caps. Combine reserved ¼ cup mushroom liquid, chicken broth, ketchup, sherry, soy sauce, vinegar and sugar in small bowl. Set aside.

2. Heat 1 teaspoon oil in large saucepan over medium heat. Add ginger and garlic; stir-fry 10 seconds. Add mushrooms, tomato and green onion; stir-fry 1 minute. Add chicken broth mixture; bring to a boil over high heat. Reduce heat to medium; simmer 10 minutes.

3. Combine 1 tablespoon water and cornstarch in small bowl; set aside. Heat remaining ½ teaspoon oil in large nonstick skillet over medium heat. Add zucchini and yellow onion; stir-fry 30 seconds. Add remaining 3 tablespoons water. Cover and cook 3 to 4 minutes or until vegetables are crisp-tender, stirring occasionally. Add tomato mixture to skillet. Stir cornstarch mixture and add to skillet. Cook until sauce boils and thickens.

Makes 4 servings

Nutrients per Serving: Calories: 72 (23% Calories from Fat), Total Fat: 2 g, Saturated Fat: trace, Protein: 3 g, Carbohydrate: 12 g, Cholesterol: 0 mg, Sodium: 156 mg, Fiber: 3 g, Sugar: 3 g
Dietary Exchanges: 2 Vegetable, 1 Fat

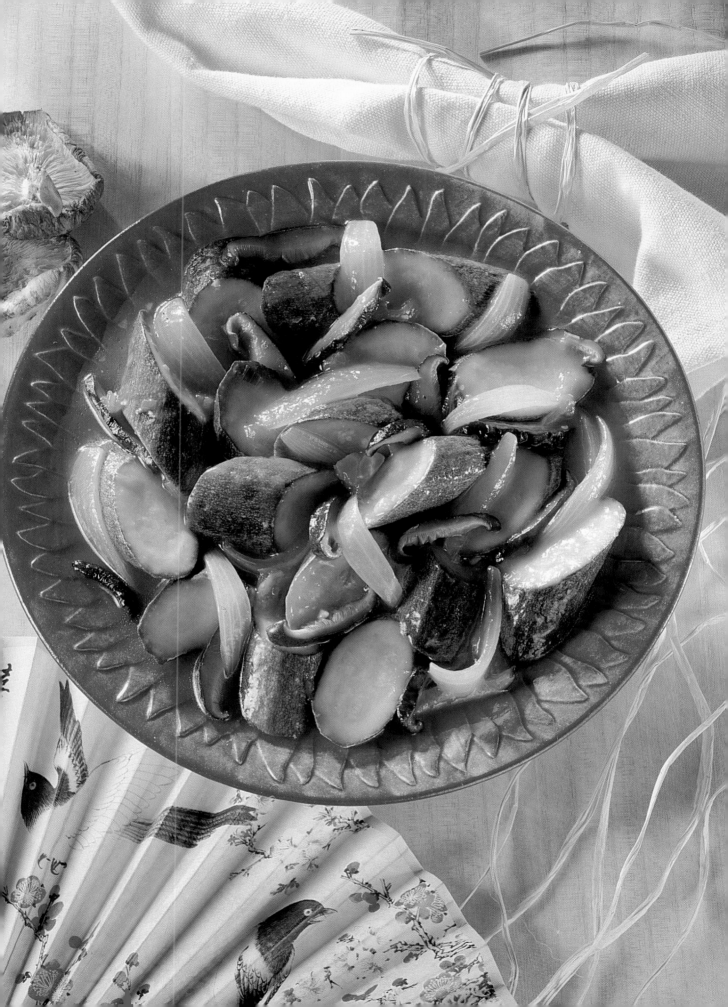

Glazed Maple Acorn Squash

Although acorn squash is considered a winter squash, it is usually available year round. Look for golden acorn squash, which is similar in all respects to the typical green acorn squash, but its shell has a dramatic pumpkin color.

1 large acorn or golden acorn squash
¼ cup water
2 tablespoons pure maple syrup
1 tablespoon margarine or butter, melted
¼ teaspoon cinnamon

1. Preheat oven to 375°F.

2. Cut stem and blossom ends from squash. Cut squash crosswise into four equal slices. Discard seeds and membrane. Place water in 13×9-inch baking dish. Arrange squash in dish; cover with foil. Bake 30 minutes or until tender.

3. Combine syrup, margarine and cinnamon in small bowl; mix well. Uncover squash; pour off water. Brush squash with syrup mixture, letting excess pool in center of squash.

4. Return to oven; bake 10 minutes or until syrup mixture is bubbly.

Makes 4 servings

Nutrients per Serving: Calories: 161 (16% Calories from Fat), Total Fat: 3 g, Saturated Fat: 2 g, Protein: 2 g, Carbohydrate: 35 g, Cholesterol: 8 mg, Sodium: 39 mg, Fiber: 4 g, Sugar: 14 g
Dietary Exchanges: 2 Starch/Bread, ½ Fat

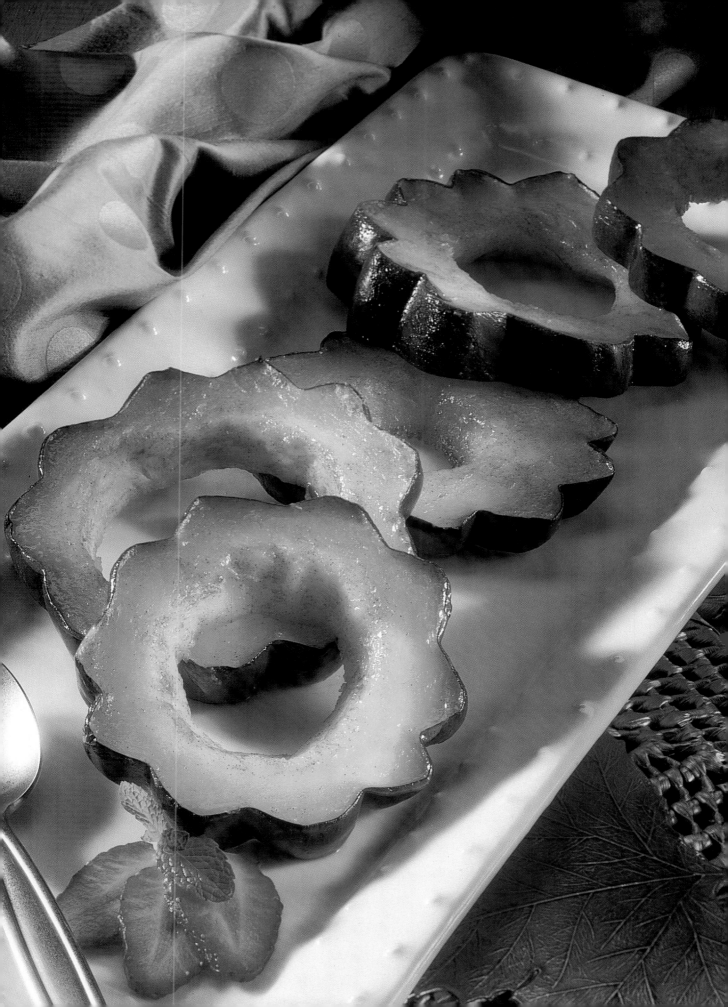

Spicy Sesame Noodles

Soba is a Japanese noodle made from buckwheat flour with a taste and texture that are different from the kind of spaghetti familiar to most Americans.

6 ounces uncooked dry soba (buckwheat) noodles
2 teaspoons dark sesame oil
1 tablespoon sesame seeds
½ cup fat-free reduced-sodium chicken broth
1 tablespoon creamy peanut butter
4 teaspoons light soy sauce
½ cup thinly sliced green onions
½ cup minced red bell pepper
1½ teaspoons finely chopped, seeded jalapeño pepper*
1 clove garlic, minced
¼ teaspoon red pepper flakes

*Jalapeño peppers can sting and irritate the skin; wear rubber gloves when handling peppers and do not touch eyes. Wash hands after handling.

1. Cook noodles according to package directions. (Do not overcook.) Rinse noodles thoroughly with cold water to stop cooking and remove salty residue; drain. Place noodles in large bowl; toss with sesame oil.

2. Place sesame seeds in small skillet. Cook over medium heat about 3 minutes or until seeds begin to pop and turn golden brown, stirring frequently. Remove from heat; set aside.

3. Combine chicken broth and peanut butter in small bowl with wire whisk until blended. (Mixture may look curdled.) Stir in soy sauce, green onions, bell pepper, jalapeño pepper, garlic and red pepper flakes.

4. Pour mixture over noodles; toss to coat. Cover and let stand 30 minutes at room temperature or refrigerate up to 24 hours. Sprinkle with toasted sesame seeds before serving.   *Makes 6 servings*

Nutrients per Serving: Calories: 145 (23% Calories from Fat), Total Fat: 4 g, Saturated Fat: 1 g, Protein: 6 g, Carbohydrate: 24 g, Cholesterol: 0 mg, Sodium: 358 mg, Fiber: 1 g, Sugar: 1 g
Dietary Exchanges: 1½ Starch/Bread, ½ Vegetable, ½ Fat

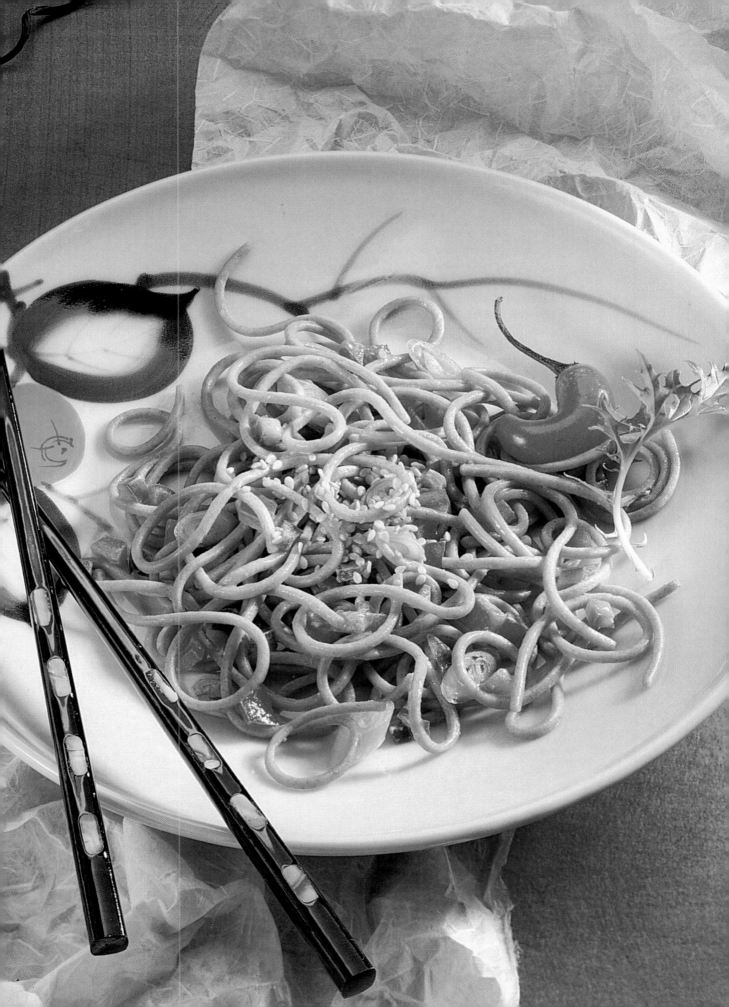

Gratin of Two Potatoes

This delicious side dish can be prepared up to 2 hours before baking. Let stand, covered with foil, at room temperature.

2 large baking potatoes (about 1¼ pounds)
2 large sweet potatoes (about 1¼ pounds)
1 tablespoon unsalted butter
1 large sweet or yellow onion, thinly sliced, separated into rings
2 teaspoons all-purpose flour
1 cup canned fat-free reduced-sodium chicken broth
½ teaspoon salt
¼ teaspoon ground white pepper *or* ⅛ teaspoon ground red pepper
¾ cup freshly grated Parmesan cheese

1. Cook baking potatoes in large pot of boiling water 10 minutes. Add sweet potatoes; return to a boil. Simmer potatoes, uncovered, 25 minutes or until tender. Drain; cool under cold running water.

2. Meanwhile, melt butter in large nonstick skillet over medium-high heat. Add onion; cover and cook 3 minutes or until wilted. Uncover; cook over medium-low heat 10 to 12 minutes or until tender, stirring occasionally. Sprinkle with flour; cook 1 minute, stirring frequently. Add chicken broth, salt and pepper; bring to a boil over high heat. Reduce heat to medium; simmer, uncovered, 2 minutes or until sauce thickens, stirring occasionally.

3. Preheat oven to 375°F. Spray 13×9-inch baking dish with nonstick cooking spray. Peel potatoes; cut crosswise into ¼-inch slices. Layer half of baking and sweet potato slices in prepared dish. Spoon half of onion mixture evenly over potatoes. Repeat layering with remaining potatoes and onion mixture. Cover with foil. Bake 25 minutes or until heated through.

4. Preheat broiler. Uncover potatoes; sprinkle evenly with cheese. Broil, 5 inches from heat, 3 to 4 minutes or until cheese is bubbly and light golden brown.   *Makes 6 servings*

Nutrients per Serving: Calories: 261 (21% Calories from Fat), Total Fat: 6 g, Saturated Fat: 4 g, Protein: 9 g, Carbohydrate: 43 g, Cholesterol: 15 mg, Sodium: 437 mg, Fiber: 1 g, Sugar: 1 g
Dietary Exchanges: 3 Starch/Bread, ½ Lean Meat, ½ Fat

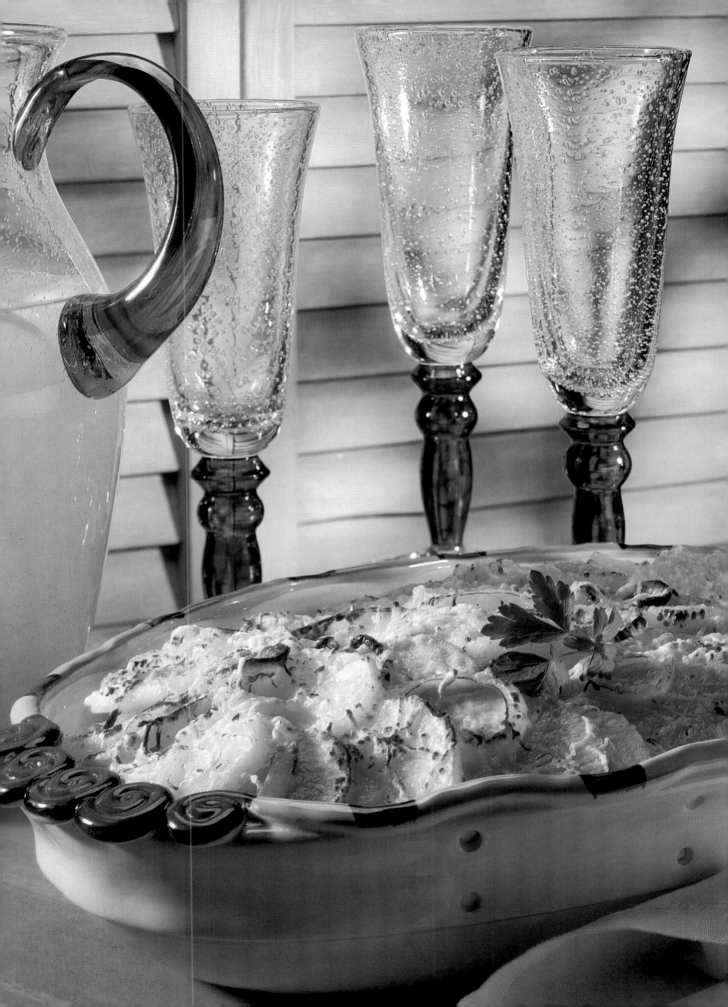

Mediterranean-Style Roasted Vegetables

This colorful side dish is a perfect accompaniment to grilled chicken or pork.

   1½ **pounds red potatoes**
   1 **tablespoon plus 1½ teaspoons olive oil, divided**
   1 **red bell pepper**
   1 **yellow or orange bell pepper**
   1 **small red onion**
   2 **cloves garlic, minced**
   ½ **teaspoon salt**
   ¼ **teaspoon black pepper**
   1 **tablespoon balsamic vinegar**
   ¼ **cup chopped fresh basil leaves**

1. Preheat oven to 425°F. Spray large shallow metal roasting pan with nonstick cooking spray. Cut potatoes into 1½-inch chunks; place in pan. Drizzle 1 tablespoon oil over potatoes; toss to coat. Bake 10 minutes.

2. Cut bell peppers into 1½-inch chunks. Cut onion through the core into ½-inch wedges. Add bell peppers and onion to pan. Drizzle remaining 1½ teaspoons oil over vegetables; sprinkle with garlic, salt and black pepper. Toss well to coat. Return to oven; bake 18 to 20 minutes or until vegetables are brown and tender, stirring once.

3. Transfer to large serving bowl. Drizzle vinegar over vegetables; toss to coat. Add basil; toss again. Serve warm or at room temperature with additional black pepper, if desired.   *Makes 6 servings*

Nutrients per Serving: Calories: 170 (19% Calories from Fat), Total Fat: 4 g, Saturated Fat: trace, Protein: 3 g, Carbohydrate: 33 g, Cholesterol: 0 mg, Sodium: 185 mg, Fiber: 1 g, Sugar: trace
Dietary Exchanges: 2 Starch/Bread, ½ Fat

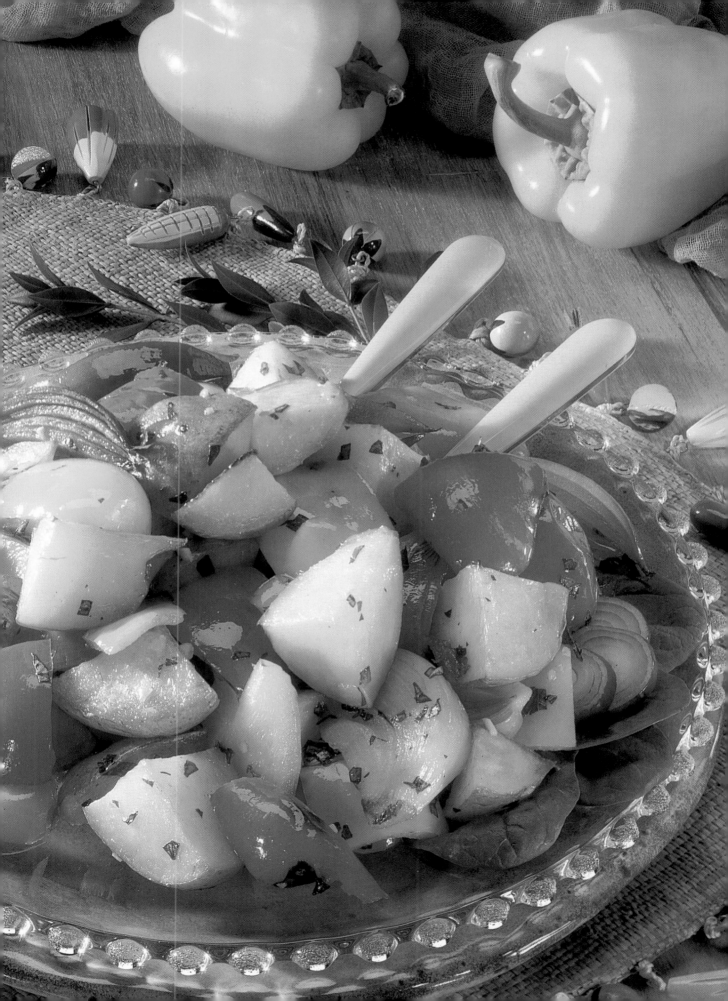

Spinach Parmesan Risotto

Arborio rice, an Italian-grown short-grain rice, has large, plump grains with a delicious nutty taste. It is traditionally used for risotto dishes because its high starch content produces a creamy texture.

3⅔ cups fat-free reduced-sodium chicken broth
½ teaspoon ground white pepper
　　Nonstick cooking spray
1 cup uncooked arborio rice
1½ cups chopped fresh spinach
½ cup frozen green peas
1 tablespoon minced fresh dill *or* **1 teaspoon dried dill weed**
½ cup grated Parmesan cheese
1 teaspoon grated lemon peel

1. Combine chicken broth and pepper in medium saucepan; cover. Bring to a simmer over medium-low heat; maintain simmer by adjusting heat.

2. Spray large saucepan with cooking spray; heat over medium-low heat. Add rice; cook and stir 1 minute. Stir in ⅔ cup hot chicken broth; cook, stirring constantly until chicken broth is absorbed.

3. Stir remaining hot chicken broth into rice mixture, ½ cup at a time, stirring constantly until all chicken broth is absorbed before adding next ½ cup. When adding last ½ cup chicken broth, stir in spinach, peas and dill. Cook, stirring gently until all chicken broth is absorbed and rice is just tender but still firm to the bite. (Total cooking time for chicken broth absorption is 35 to 40 minutes.)

4. Remove saucepan from heat; stir in cheese and lemon peel.

Makes 6 servings

Nutrients per Serving: Calories: 179 (15% Calories from Fat), Total Fat: 3 g, Saturated Fat: 2 g, Protein: 7 g, Carbohydrate: 30 g, Cholesterol: 7 mg, Sodium: 198 mg, Fiber: 1 g, Sugar: 1 g
Dietary Exchanges: 2 Starch/Bread, ½ Lean Meat

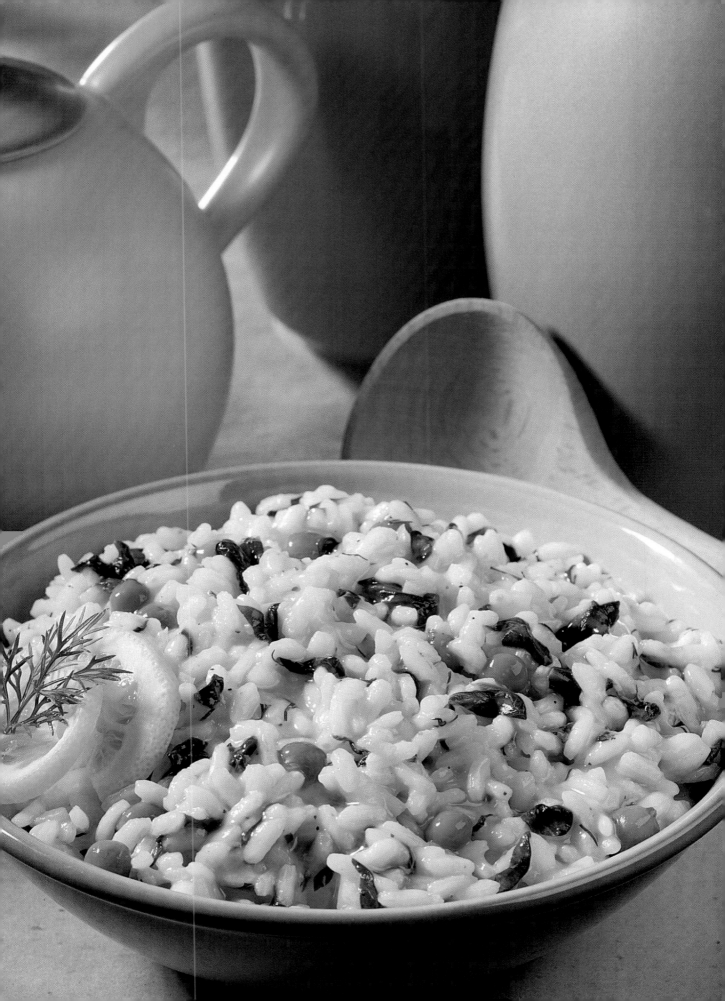

Main Dishes

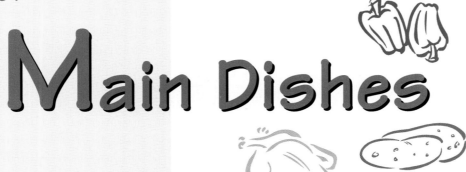

Roast Chicken & Potatoes Catalan

- 2 tablespoons olive oil
- 2 tablespoons lemon juice
- 1 teaspoon dried thyme leaves
- ½ teaspoon salt
- ¼ teaspoon ground red pepper
- ¼ teaspoon ground saffron *or* ½ teaspoon crushed saffron threads or turmeric
- 2 large baking potatoes (about 1½ pounds), cut into 1½-inch chunks
- 4 skinless bone-in chicken breast halves (about 2 pounds)
- 1 cup sliced red bell pepper
- 1 cup frozen peas, thawed
- Lemon wedges

1. Preheat oven to 400°F. Spray large shallow roasting pan or 15×10-inch jelly-roll pan with nonstick cooking spray.

2. Combine oil, lemon juice, thyme, salt, ground red pepper and saffron in large bowl; mix well. Add potatoes; toss to coat.

3. Arrange potatoes in single layer around edges of pan. Place chicken in center of pan; brush both sides of chicken with remaining oil mixture in bowl.

4. Bake 20 minutes. Turn potatoes; baste chicken with pan juices. Add bell pepper; continue baking 20 minutes or until chicken is no longer pink in center, juices run clear and potatoes are browned. Stir peas into potato mixture; bake 5 minutes or until heated through. Garnish with lemon wedges.

Makes 4 servings

Nutrients per Serving: Calories: 541 (18% Calories from Fat), Total Fat: 11 g, Saturated Fat: 2 g, Protein: 42 g, Carbohydrate: 69 g, Cholesterol: 91 mg, Sodium: 132 mg, Fiber: 3 g, Sugar: 2 g
Dietary Exchanges: 4 Starch/Bread, 4 Lean Meat, 1 Vegetable

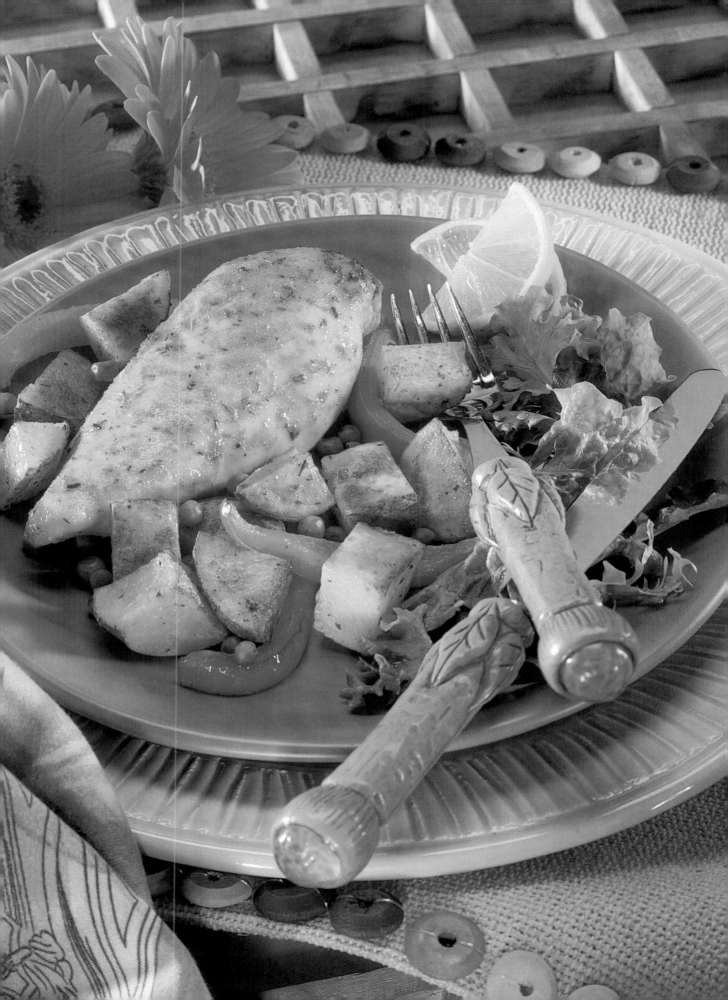

Mushroom Ragoût with Polenta

This easy meatless main dish will please the whole family. Cooking the polenta in the microwave oven is foolproof and makes cleanup easy.

1 package (about ½ ounce) dried porcini mushrooms
½ cup boiling water
1 can (about 14 ounces) vegetable broth
½ cup yellow cornmeal
1 tablespoon olive oil
⅓ cup sliced shallots or chopped sweet onion
1 package (4 ounces) sliced mixed fresh exotic mushrooms or sliced cremini mushrooms
4 cloves garlic, minced
1 can (14½ ounces) Italian-style diced tomatoes, undrained
¼ teaspoon red pepper flakes
¼ cup chopped fresh basil or parsley
½ cup grated fat-free Parmesan cheese

1. Soak porcini mushrooms in boiling water 10 minutes.

2. Meanwhile, whisk together vegetable broth and cornmeal in large microwavable bowl. Cover with waxed paper; microwave at HIGH 5 minutes. Whisk well; cook at HIGH 3 to 4 minutes or until polenta is very thick. Whisk again; cover. Set aside.

3. Heat oil in large nonstick skillet over medium-high heat. Add shallots; cook and stir 3 minutes. Add fresh mushrooms and garlic; cook and stir 3 to 4 minutes. Add tomatoes and red pepper flakes.

4. Drain porcini mushrooms; add liquid to skillet. If mushrooms are large, cut into ½-inch pieces; add to skillet. Bring to a boil over high heat. Reduce heat to medium; simmer, uncovered, 5 minutes or until slightly thickened. Stir in basil.

5. Spoon polenta onto 4 plates; top with mushroom mixture. Sprinkle with cheese.   *Makes 4 servings*

Nutrients per Serving: Calories: 184 (25% Calories from Fat), Total Fat: 5 g, Saturated Fat: 1 g, Protein: 6 g, Carbohydrate: 30 g, Cholesterol: 0 mg, Sodium: 572 mg, Fiber: 3 g, Sugar: 6 g
Dietary Exchanges: 1 Starch/Bread, ½ Lean Meat, 2½ Vegetable, ½ Fat

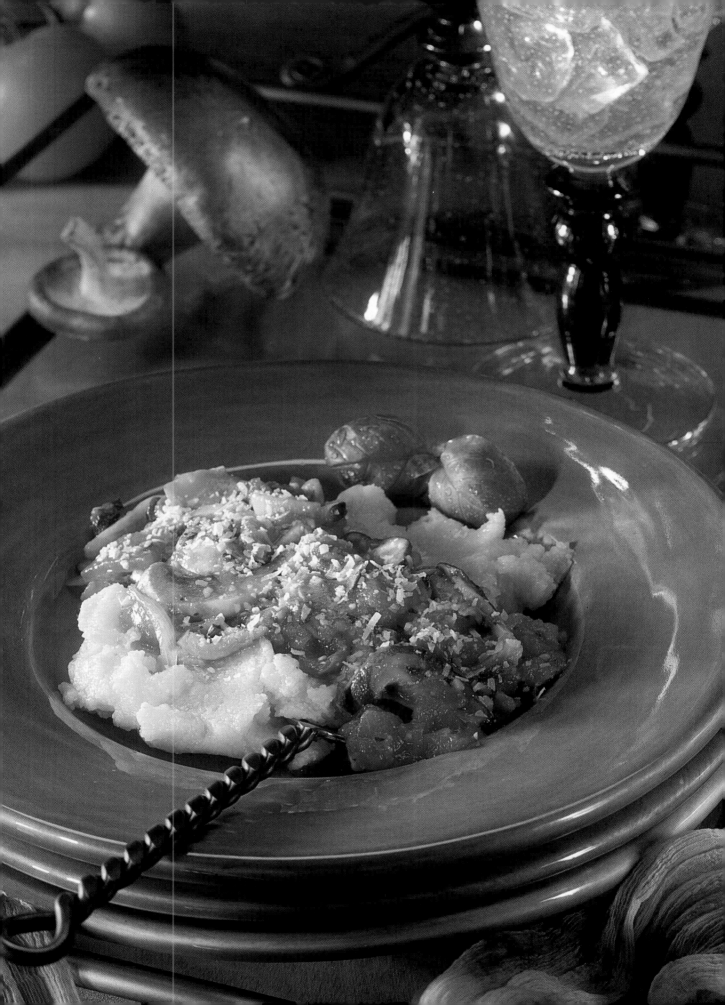

Thai-Style Pork Kabobs

Wooden skewers may be substituted for metal skewers. Soak them in cold water for 20 minutes to prevent them from burning during grilling.

- **⅓ cup reduced-sodium soy sauce**
- **2 tablespoons fresh lime juice**
- **2 tablespoons water**
- **2 teaspoons hot chili oil***
- **2 cloves garlic, minced**
- **1 teaspoon minced fresh ginger**
- **12 ounces well-trimmed pork tenderloin**
- **1 red or yellow bell pepper, cut into ½-inch chunks**
- **1 red or sweet onion, cut into ½-inch chunks**
- **2 cups hot cooked rice**

*If hot chili oil is not available, combine 2 teaspoons vegetable oil and ½ teaspoon red pepper flakes in small microwavable cup. Microwave at HIGH 1 minute. Let stand 5 minutes to infuse flavor.

1. Combine soy sauce, lime juice, water, chili oil, garlic and ginger in medium bowl; reserve ⅓ cup mixture for dipping sauce. Set aside.

2. Cut pork tenderloin lengthwise in half; cut crosswise into 4-inch slices. Cut slices into ½-inch strips. Add to bowl with soy sauce mixture; toss to coat. Cover; refrigerate at least 30 minutes or up to 2 hours, turning once.

3. To prevent sticking, spray grid with nonstick cooking spray. Prepare coals for grilling.

4. Remove pork from marinade; discard marinade. Alternately weave pork strips and thread bell pepper and onion chunks onto eight 8- to 10-inch metal skewers.

5. Grill, covered, over medium-hot coals 6 to 8 minutes or until pork is no longer pink in center, turning halfway through grilling time. Serve with rice and reserved dipping sauce.   *Makes 4 servings*

Nutrients per Serving: Calories: 248 (16% Calories from Fat), Total Fat: 4 g, Saturated Fat: 1 g, Protein: 22 g, Carbohydrate: 30 g, Cholesterol: 49 mg, Sodium: 271 mg, Fiber: 2 g, Sugar: 1 g
Dietary Exchanges: 1½ Starch/Bread, 2 Lean Meat, 1 Vegetable

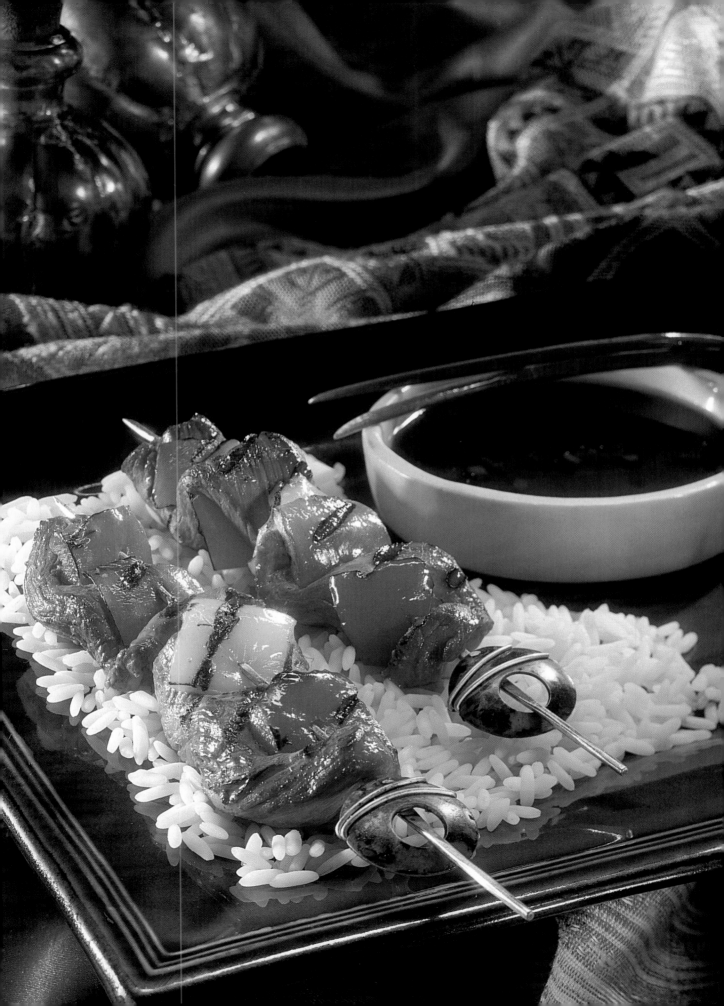

Szechwan Beef Lo Mein

Serve this spicy Asian one-dish meal with a chilled cucumber salad and fresh pineapple spears. Partially freezing the steak makes it easier to cut into strips.

>   1 pound well-trimmed boneless beef top sirloin steak, 1 inch thick
>   4 cloves garlic, minced
>   2 teaspoons minced fresh ginger
>   ¾ teaspoon red pepper flakes, divided
>   1 tablespoon vegetable oil
>   1 can (about 14 ounces) vegetable broth
>   1 cup water
>   2 tablespoons reduced-sodium soy sauce
>   1 package (8 ounces) frozen mixed vegetables for stir-fry
>   1 package (9 ounces) refrigerated angel hair pasta
>   ¼ cup chopped cilantro (optional)

1. Cut steak crosswise into ⅛-inch strips; cut strips into 1½-inch pieces. Toss steak with garlic, ginger and ½ teaspoon red pepper flakes.

2. Heat oil in large nonstick skillet over medium-high heat. Add half of steak to skillet; cook and stir 3 minutes or until meat is barely pink in center. Remove from skillet; set aside. Repeat with remaining steak.

3. Add vegetable broth, water, soy sauce and remaining ¼ teaspoon red pepper flakes to skillet; bring to a boil over high heat. Add vegetables; return to a boil. Reduce heat to low; simmer, covered, 3 minutes or until vegetables are crisp-tender.

4. Uncover; stir in pasta. Return to a boil over high heat. Reduce heat to medium; simmer, uncovered, 2 minutes, separating pasta with two forks. Return steak and any accumulated juices to skillet; simmer 1 minute or until pasta is tender and steak is hot. Sprinkle with cilantro, if desired.

Makes 4 servings

Nutrients per Serving: Calories: 408 (25% Calories from Fat), Total Fat: 11 g, Saturated Fat: 3 g, Protein: 32 g, Carbohydrate: 44 g, Cholesterol: 137 mg, Sodium: 386 mg, Fiber: 2 g, Sugar: 1 g
Dietary Exchanges: 2 Starch/Bread, 3 Lean Meat, 3 Vegetable, ½ Fat

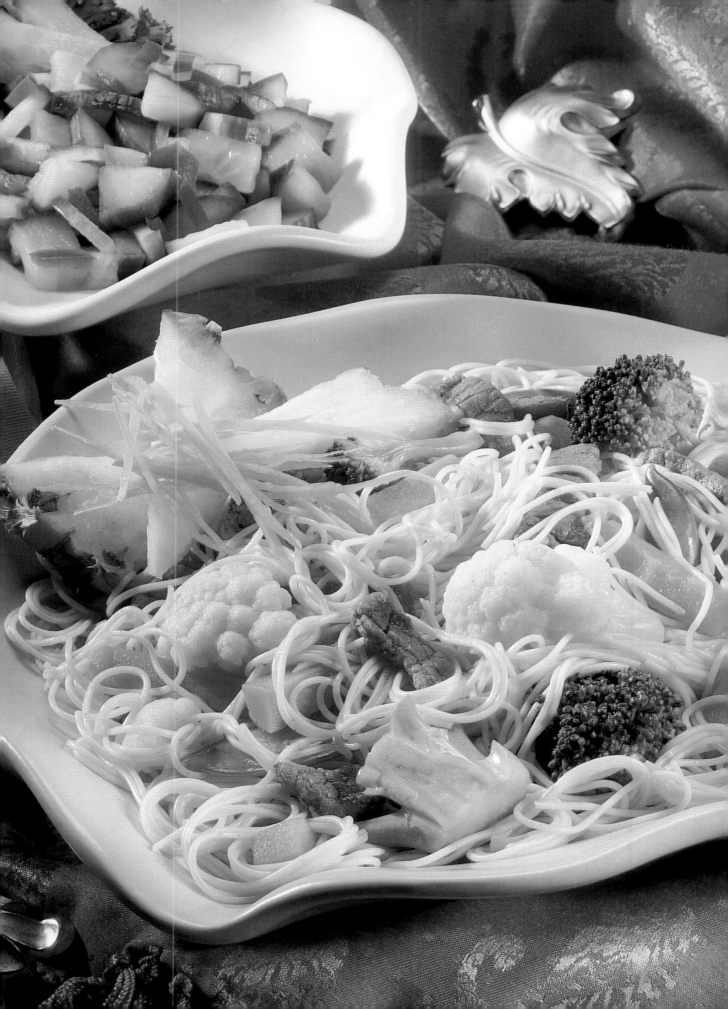

Broiled Caribbean Sea Bass

This flavorful fish entrée needs only 30 minutes to marinate and cooks quickly. The black bean and rice mix provides a quick yet authentic accompaniment to the fish.

6 skinless sea bass or striped bass fillets (5 to 6 ounces each), about ½ inch thick
⅓ cup chopped cilantro
2 tablespoons olive oil
2 tablespoons fresh lime juice
2 teaspoons hot pepper sauce
2 cloves garlic, minced
1 package (7 ounces) black bean and rice mix
Lime wedges

1. Place fish in shallow dish. Combine cilantro, oil, lime juice, pepper sauce and garlic in small bowl; pour over fish. Cover; marinate in refrigerator 30 minutes or up to 2 hours.

2. Prepare black bean and rice mix according to package directions; keep warm.

3. Preheat broiler. Remove fish from marinade. Place fish on rack of broiler pan; drizzle with any remaining marinade in dish. Broil, 4 to 5 inches from heat, 8 to 10 minutes or until fish is opaque. Serve with black beans and rice and lime wedges.   *Makes 6 servings*

Nutrients per Serving: Calories: 307 (23% Calories from Fat), Total Fat: 8 g, Saturated Fat: 1 g, Protein: 33 g, Carbohydrate: 30 g, Cholesterol: 59 mg, Sodium: 432 mg, Fiber: 5 g, Sugar: 5 g
Dietary Exchanges: 2 Starch/Bread, 3 Lean Meat

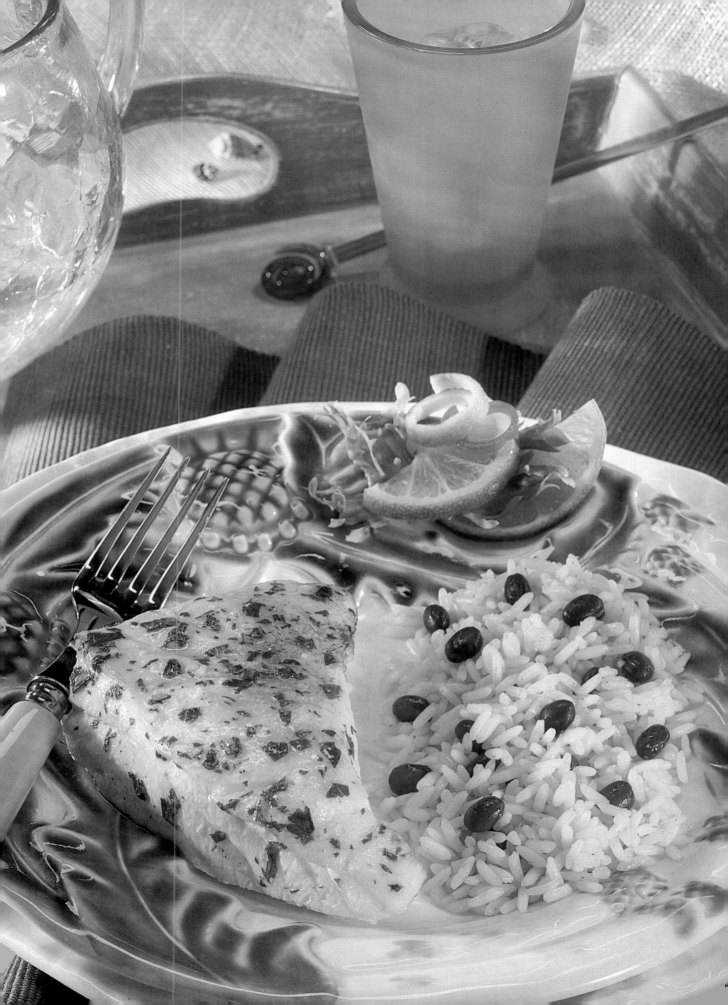

Curried Chicken & Vegetables with Rice

Serve this spicy curry with traditional condiments of toasted coconut and mango chutney.

- **1 pound chicken tenders or boneless skinless chicken breasts, cut crosswise into ½-inch slices**
- **2 teaspoons curry powder**
- **¼ teaspoon ground red pepper**
- **¼ teaspoon salt**
- **1 tablespoon vegetable oil**
- **1 medium onion, chopped**
- **3 cloves garlic, minced**
- **1¼ cups canned fat-free reduced-sodium chicken broth, divided**
- **2 tablespoons tomato paste**
- **1 package (16 ounces) frozen mixed vegetable medley, such as broccoli, red bell peppers, cauliflower and sugar snap peas, thawed**
- **2 teaspoons cornstarch**
- **3 cups hot cooked white rice**
- **½ cup plain nonfat yogurt**
- **⅓ cup chopped cilantro**

1. Toss chicken with curry powder, ground red pepper and salt in medium bowl; set aside.

2. Heat oil in large skillet over medium heat. Add onion; cook 5 minutes, stirring occasionally. Add chicken and garlic; cook 4 minutes or until chicken is no longer pink in center, stirring occasionally. Add 1 cup chicken broth, tomato paste and vegetables; bring to a boil over high heat. Reduce heat to medium; simmer, uncovered, 3 to 4 minutes or until vegetables are crisp-tender.

3. Combine remaining ¼ cup chicken broth and cornstarch, mixing until smooth. Stir into chicken mixture; simmer 2 minutes or until sauce thickens, stirring occasionally. Serve over rice; top with yogurt and cilantro.   *Makes 4 servings*

Nutrients per Serving: Calories: 404 (16% Calories from Fat), Total Fat: 7 g, Saturated Fat: 1 g, Protein: 34 g, Carbohydrate: 50 g, Cholesterol: 69 mg, Sodium: 299 mg, Fiber: 4 g, Sugar: 2 g
Dietary Exchanges: 2½ Starch/Bread, 3 Lean Meat, 2 Vegetable

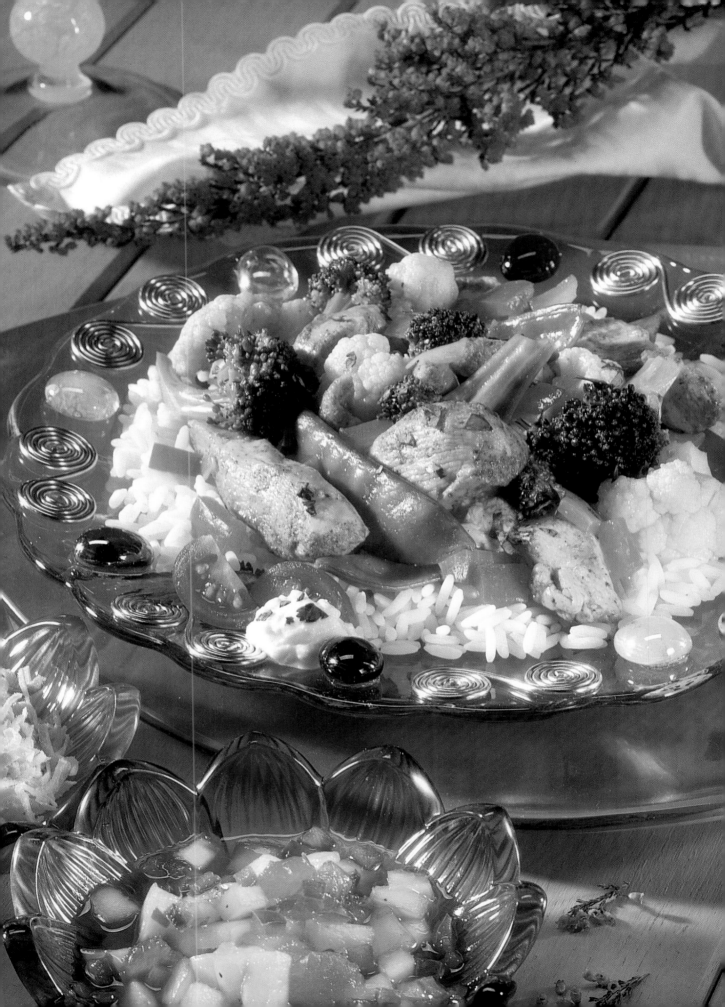

Chipotle Tamale Pie

Chipotle chilies are smoked jalapeño peppers. Look for cans of smoky hot chipotle chilies in the ethnic section of your supermarket.

¾ pound ground turkey breast or lean ground beef
1 cup chopped onion
¾ cup diced green bell pepper
¾ cup diced red bell pepper
4 cloves garlic, minced
2 teaspoons ground cumin
1 can (15 ounces) pinto or red beans, rinsed and drained
1 can (8 ounces) no-salt-added stewed tomatoes, undrained
2 canned chipotle chilies in adobo sauce, minced (about 1 tablespoon)
1 to 2 teaspoons adobo sauce from canned chilies (optional)
1 cup (4 ounces) low-sodium reduced-fat shredded Cheddar cheese
½ cup chopped cilantro
1 package (8½ ounces) corn bread mix
⅓ cup 1% low-fat milk
1 large egg white

1. Preheat oven to 400°F.

2. Cook turkey, onion, bell peppers and garlic in large nonstick skillet over medium-high heat 8 minutes or until turkey is no longer pink, stirring occasionally. Drain fat; sprinkle mixture with cumin.

3. Add beans, tomatoes, chilies and adobo sauce; bring to a boil over high heat. Reduce heat to medium; simmer, uncovered, 5 minutes. Remove from heat; stir in cheese and cilantro.

4. Spray 8-inch square baking dish with nonstick cooking spray. Spoon turkey mixture evenly into prepared dish, pressing down to compact mixture. Combine corn bread mix, milk and egg white in medium bowl; mix just until dry ingredients are moistened. Spoon batter evenly over turkey mixture to cover completely.

5. Bake 20 to 22 minutes or until corn bread is golden brown. Let stand 5 minutes before serving.   *Makes 6 servings*

Nutrients per Serving: Calories: 396 (23% Calories from Fat), Total Fat: 10 g, Saturated Fat: 3 g, Protein: 26 g, Carbohydrate: 52 g, Cholesterol: 32 mg, Sodium: 733 mg, Fiber: 2 g, Sugar: 3 g
Dietary Exchanges: 3 Starch/Bread, 2 Lean Meat, 1½ Vegetable, ½ Fat

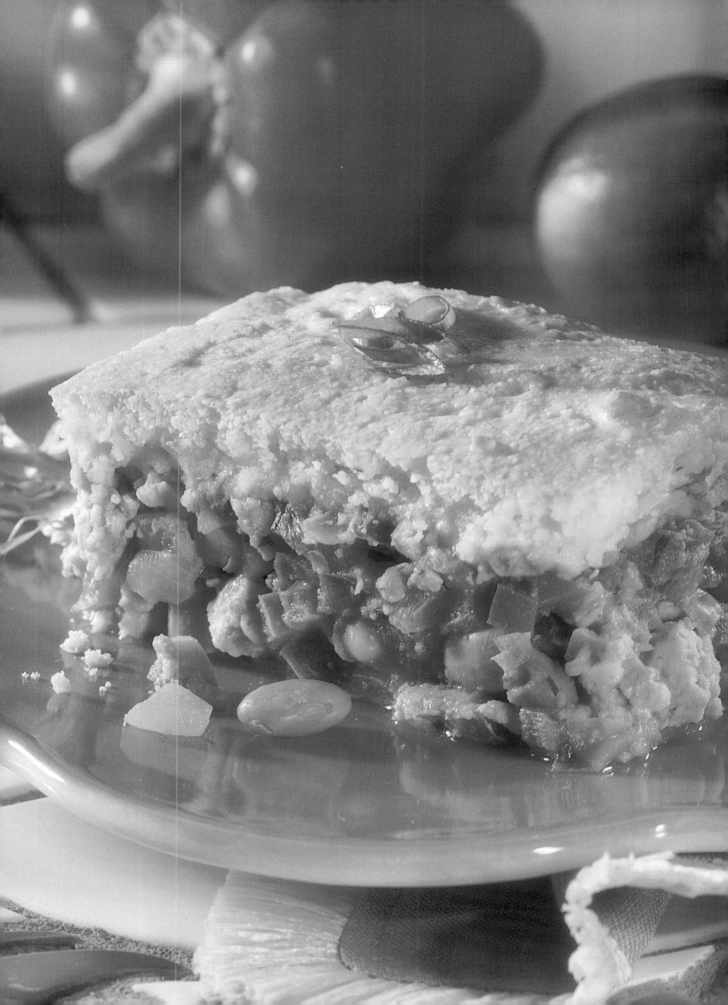

Latin-Style Pasta & Beans

Round out this hearty meatless main dish with warm corn tortillas and slices of melon.

8 ounces uncooked mostaccioli, penne or bow tie pasta
1 tablespoon olive oil
1 medium onion, chopped
1 yellow or red bell pepper, diced
4 cloves garlic, minced
1 can (15 ounces) red or black beans, rinsed and drained
¾ cup canned vegetable broth
¾ cup medium-hot salsa or picante sauce
2 teaspoons ground cumin
⅓ cup coarsely chopped cilantro
Lime wedges

1. Cook pasta according to package directions, omitting salt. Drain; set aside.

2. Meanwhile, heat oil in a large skillet over medium heat. Add onion; cook 5 minutes, stirring occasionally. Add bell pepper and garlic; cook 3 minutes, stirring occasionally. Add beans, vegetable broth, salsa and cumin; simmer, uncovered, 5 minutes.

3. Add pasta to skillet; cook 1 minute, tossing frequently. Stir in cilantro; spoon onto 4 plates. Serve with lime wedges.   *Makes 4 servings*

Nutrients per Serving: Calories: 390 (12% Calories from Fat), Total Fat: 6 g, Saturated Fat: 1 g, Protein: 18 g, Carbohydrate: 74 g, Cholesterol: 0 mg, Sodium: 557 mg, Fiber: 8 g, Sugar: 1 g
Dietary Exchanges: 4 Starch/Bread, 1 Lean Meat, 1 Vegetable, ½ Fat

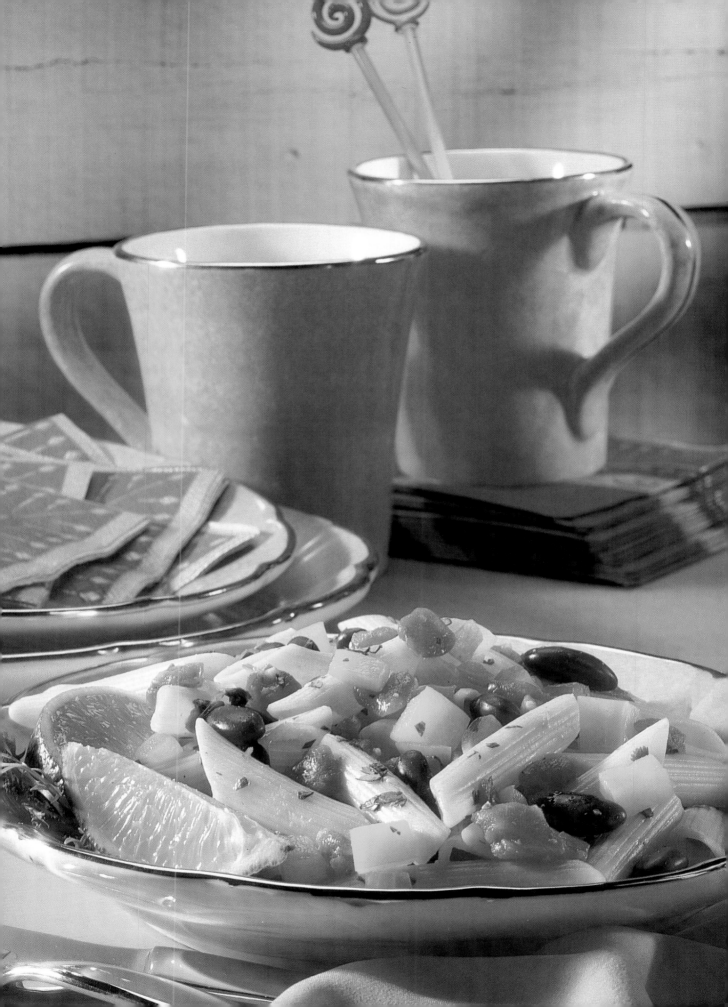

Moroccan Pork Tagine

Tagine is a traditional Moroccan stew typically made with chicken or lamb, vegetables and spices that is served over couscous. This tagine features pork tenderloin, which is naturally very lean and flavorful.

   1 pound well-trimmed pork tenderloin, cut into ¾-inch medallions
   1 tablespoon all-purpose flour
   1 teaspoon ground cumin
   1 teaspoon paprika
  ¼ teaspoon powdered saffron *or* ½ teaspoon turmeric
  ¼ teaspoon ground red pepper
  ¼ teaspoon ground ginger
   1 tablespoon olive oil
   1 medium onion, chopped
   3 cloves garlic, minced
 2½ cups canned chicken broth, divided
  ⅓ cup golden or dark raisins
   1 cup quick-cooking couscous
  ¼ cup chopped cilantro
  ¼ cup sliced toasted almonds (optional)

1. Toss pork with flour, cumin, paprika, saffron, pepper and ginger in medium bowl; set aside.

2. Heat oil in large nonstick skillet over medium-high heat. Add onion; cook 5 minutes, stirring occasionally. Add pork and garlic; cook 4 to 5 minutes or until pork is no longer pink, stirring occasionally. Add ¾ cup chicken broth and raisins; bring to a boil over high heat. Reduce heat to medium; simmer, uncovered, 7 to 8 minutes or until pork is cooked through, stirring occasionally.

3. Meanwhile, bring remaining 1¾ cups chicken broth to a boil in medium saucepan. Stir in couscous. Cover; remove from heat. Let stand 5 minutes or until liquid is absorbed.

4. Spoon couscous onto 4 plates; top with pork mixture. Sprinkle with cilantro and almonds, if desired.   *Makes 4 servings*

Nutrients per Serving: Calories: 435 (20% Calories from Fat), Total Fat: 10 g, Saturated Fat: 2 g, Protein: 33 g, Carbohydrate: 53 g, Cholesterol: 70 mg, Sodium: 686 mg, Fiber: 8 g, Sugar: 10 g
Dietary Exchanges: 2½ Starch/Bread, 3½ Lean Meat, 1 Fruit

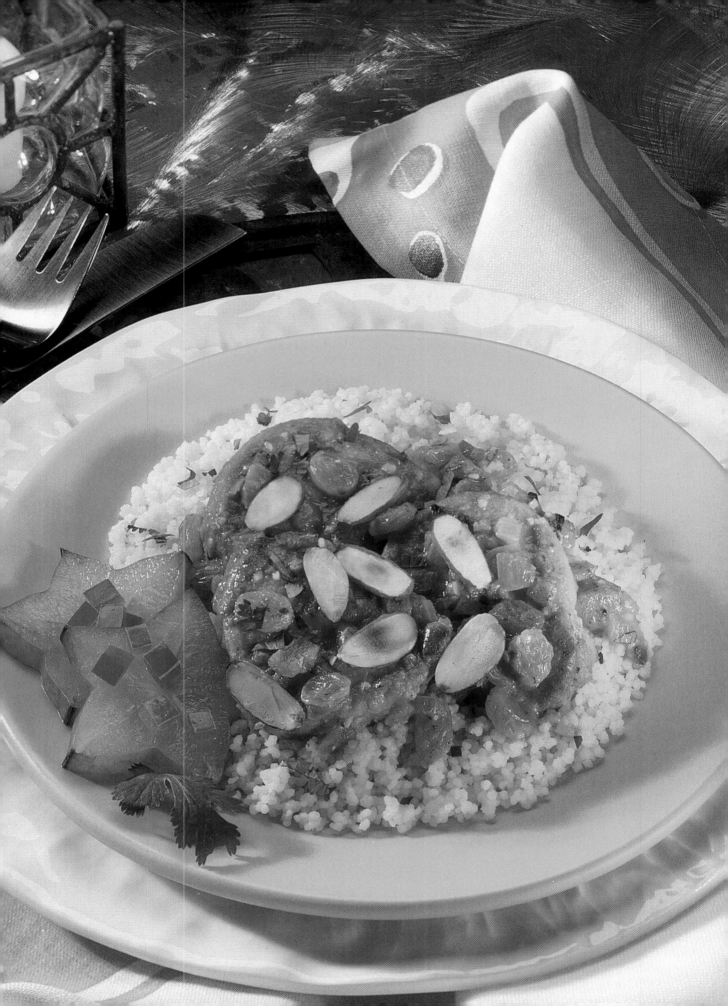

Spicy Shrimp Puttanesca

To save time, look for frozen peeled uncooked shrimp in the frozen food section of your supermarket.

8 ounces uncooked linguine, capellini or spaghetti
1 tablespoon olive oil
12 ounces medium shrimp, peeled and deveined
4 cloves garlic, minced
¾ teaspoon red pepper flakes
1 cup finely chopped onion
1 can (14½ ounces) no-salt-added stewed tomatoes, undrained
2 tablespoons tomato paste
2 tablespoons chopped pitted calamata or black olives
1 tablespoon drained capers
¼ cup chopped fresh basil or parsley

1. Cook linguine according to package directions, omitting salt. Drain; set aside.

2. Meanwhile, heat oil in large nonstick skillet over medium high heat. Add shrimp, garlic and red pepper flakes; cook and stir 3 to 4 minutes or until shrimp are opaque. Transfer shrimp mixture to bowl with slotted spoon; set aside.

3. Add onion to same skillet; cook over medium heat 5 minutes, stirring occasionally. Add tomatoes, tomato paste, olives and capers; simmer, uncovered, 5 minutes.

4. Return shrimp mixture to skillet; simmer 1 minute. Stir in basil; simmer 1 minute. Place linguine in large serving bowl; top with shrimp mixture.

Makes 4 servings

Nutrients per Serving: Calories: 328 (22% Calories from Fat), Total Fat: 8 g, Saturated Fat: 1 g, Protein: 24 g, Carbohydrate: 42 g, Cholesterol: 131 mg, Sodium: 537 mg, Fiber: 2 g, Sugar: 4 g
Dietary Exchanges: 2 Starch/Bread, 1½ Lean Meat, 2 Vegetable, 1 Fat

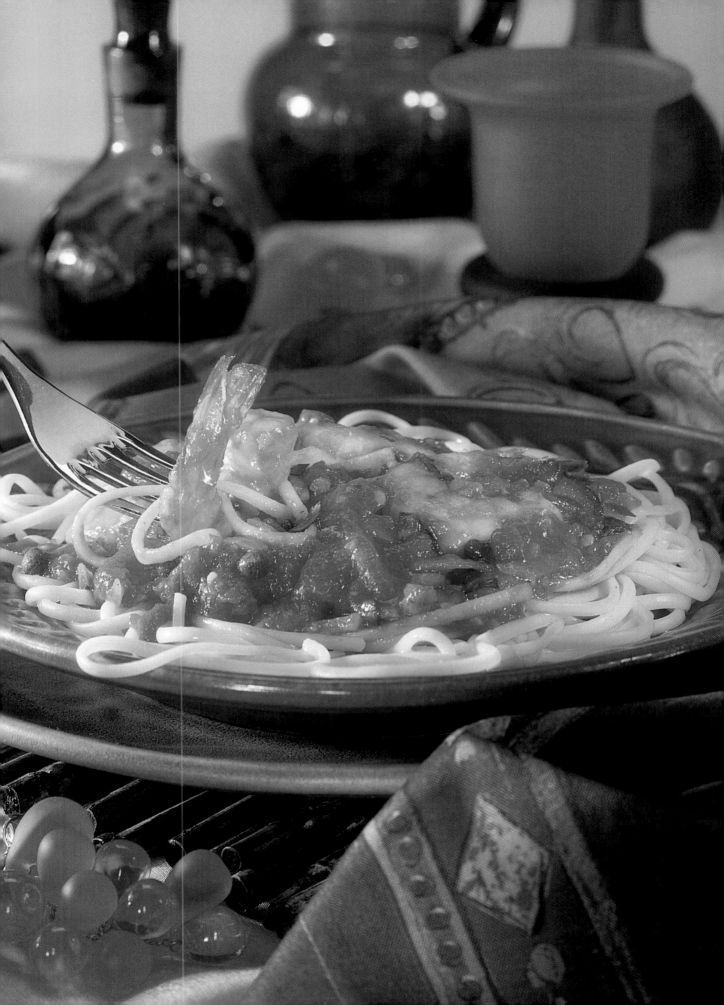

Cajun-Style Chicken Gumbo

1 pound boneless skinless chicken breasts
1 teaspoon Cajun or Creole seasoning
1 teaspoon dried thyme leaves
2 tablespoons vegetable oil
1 medium onion, coarsely chopped
1 green bell pepper, coarsely chopped
1 cup thinly sliced or julienned carrots
½ cup thinly sliced celery
4 cloves garlic, minced
2 tablespoons all-purpose flour
1 can (about 14 ounces) fat-free reduced-sodium chicken broth
1 can (14½ ounces) no-salt-added stewed tomatoes, undrained
½ teaspoon hot pepper sauce
2 cups hot cooked rice
¼ cup chopped parsley (optional)
Additional hot pepper sauce (optional)

1. Cut chicken into 1-inch pieces; place in medium bowl. Sprinkle with seasoning and thyme; toss well. Set aside.

2. Heat oil in large saucepan over medium-high heat. Add onion, bell pepper, carrots, celery and garlic to saucepan; cover and cook 10 minutes or until vegetables are crisp-tender, stirring once. Add chicken; cook 3 minutes, stirring occasionally. Sprinkle mixture with flour; cook 1 minute, stirring frequently.

3. Add chicken broth, tomatoes and pepper sauce; bring to a boil over high heat. Reduce heat to medium; simmer, uncovered, 10 minutes or until chicken is no longer pink in center, vegetables are tender and sauce is slightly thickened.

4. Ladle gumbo into 4 shallow bowls; top each with a scoop of rice. Sprinkle with parsley and serve with additional pepper sauce, if desired.

Makes 4 servings

Nutrients per Serving: Calories: 378 (26% Calories from Fat), Total Fat: 11 g, Saturated Fat: 2 g, Protein: 31 g, Carbohydrate: 39 g, Cholesterol: 69 mg, Sodium: 176 mg, Fiber: 3 g, Sugar: 6 g
Dietary Exchanges: 2 Starch/Bread, 3 Lean Meat, 2 Vegetable, ½ Fat

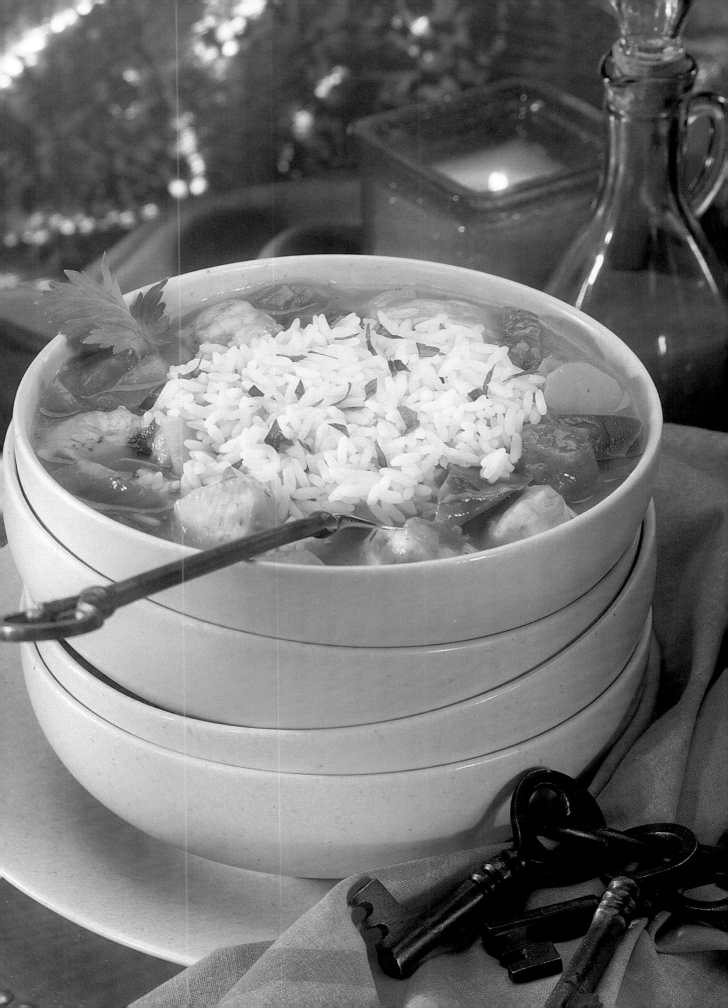

Fresh Vegetable Lasagna

8 ounces uncooked lasagna noodles
1 package (10 ounces) frozen chopped spinach, thawed and squeezed dry
1 cup shredded carrots
½ cup sliced green onions
½ cup sliced red bell pepper
¼ cup chopped parsley
½ teaspoon black pepper
1½ cups 1% low-fat cottage cheese
1 cup buttermilk
½ cup plain nonfat yogurt
2 egg whites
1 cup sliced mushrooms
1 can (14 ounces) artichoke hearts, drained and chopped
2 cups (8 ounces) shredded part-skim mozzarella cheese
¼ cup grated Parmesan cheese

1. Cook pasta according to package directions, omitting salt. Drain. Rinse under cold water until cool; drain well. Set aside.

2. Preheat oven to 375°F. Combine spinach, carrots, green onions, bell pepper, parsley and black pepper in large bowl. Set aside.

3. Combine cottage cheese, buttermilk, yogurt and egg whites in food processor or blender; process until smooth.

4. Spray 13×9-inch baking pan with nonstick cooking spray. Arrange ⅓ of lasagna noodles in bottom of pan. Spread with half *each* of cottage cheese mixture, spinach mixture, mushrooms, artichokes and mozzarella. Repeat layers, ending with noodles. Sprinkle with Parmesan cheese.

5. Cover and bake 30 minutes. Remove cover; continue baking 20 minutes or until bubbling and heated through. Let stand 10 minutes before serving.

Makes 8 servings

Nutrients per Serving: Calories: 250 (26% Calories from Fat), Total Fat: 8 g, Saturated Fat: 4 g, Protein: 22 g, Carbohydrate: 26 g, Cholesterol: 22 mg, Sodium: 508 mg, Fiber: 5 g, Sugar: 6 g
Dietary Exchanges: 1 Starch/Bread, 2 Lean Meat, 2 Vegetable, ½ Fat

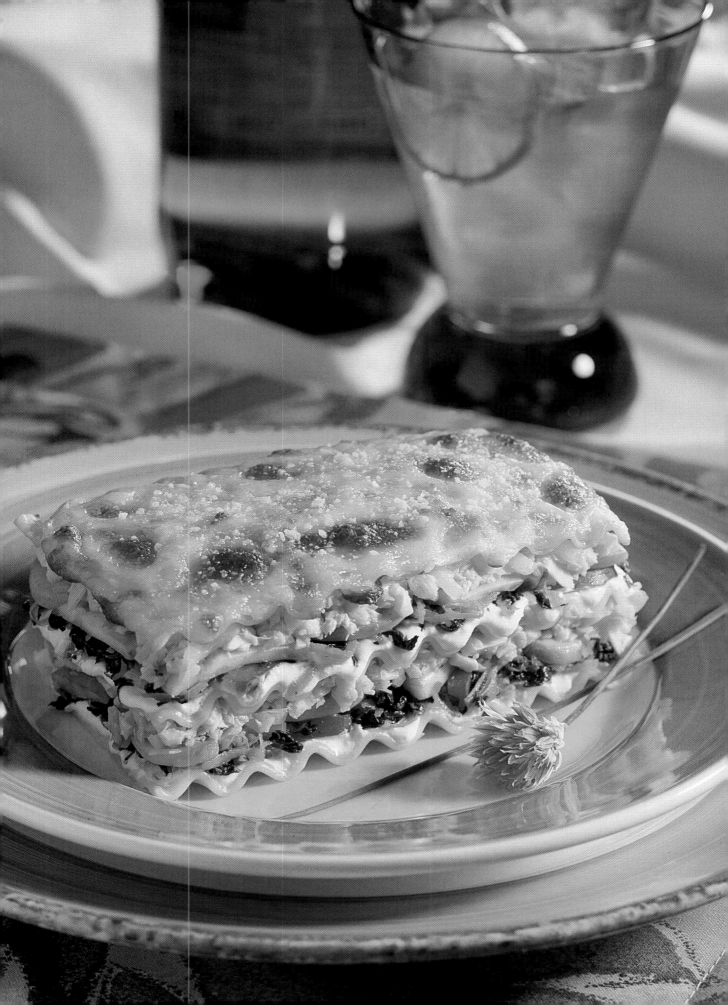

Beef & Bean Burritos

Steak plays a supporting role in these easy-to-make burritos. It's the bold flavors of cilantro and green chilies that capture the essence of Mexican cuisine.

Nonstick cooking spray
½ pound beef top round steak, cut into ½-inch strips
3 cloves garlic, minced
1 can (about 15 ounces) pinto beans, rinsed and drained
1 can (4 ounces) diced mild green chilies, drained
¼ cup finely chopped cilantro
6 (6-inch) flour tortillas
½ cup (2 ounces) shredded reduced-fat Cheddar cheese
Salsa (optional)
Nonfat sour cream (optional)

1. Spray nonstick skillet with cooking spray; heat over medium heat. Add steak and garlic; cook and stir 5 minutes or to desired doneness.

2. Add beans, chilies and cilantro; cook and stir 5 minutes or until heated through.

3. Spoon steak mixture evenly down center of each tortilla; sprinkle cheese evenly over each tortilla. Fold bottom of each tortilla up over filling, then fold sides over filling. Garnish with salsa and nonfat sour cream, if desired.   *Makes 6 servings*

Nutrients per Serving: Calories: 278 (22% Calories from Fat), Total Fat: 7 g, Saturated Fat: 2 g, Protein: 19 g, Carbohydrate: 36 g, Cholesterol: 31 mg, Sodium: 956 mg, Fiber: 1 g, Sugar: trace
Dietary Exchanges: 2 Starch/Bread, 1½ Lean Meat, 1 Vegetable, ½ Fat

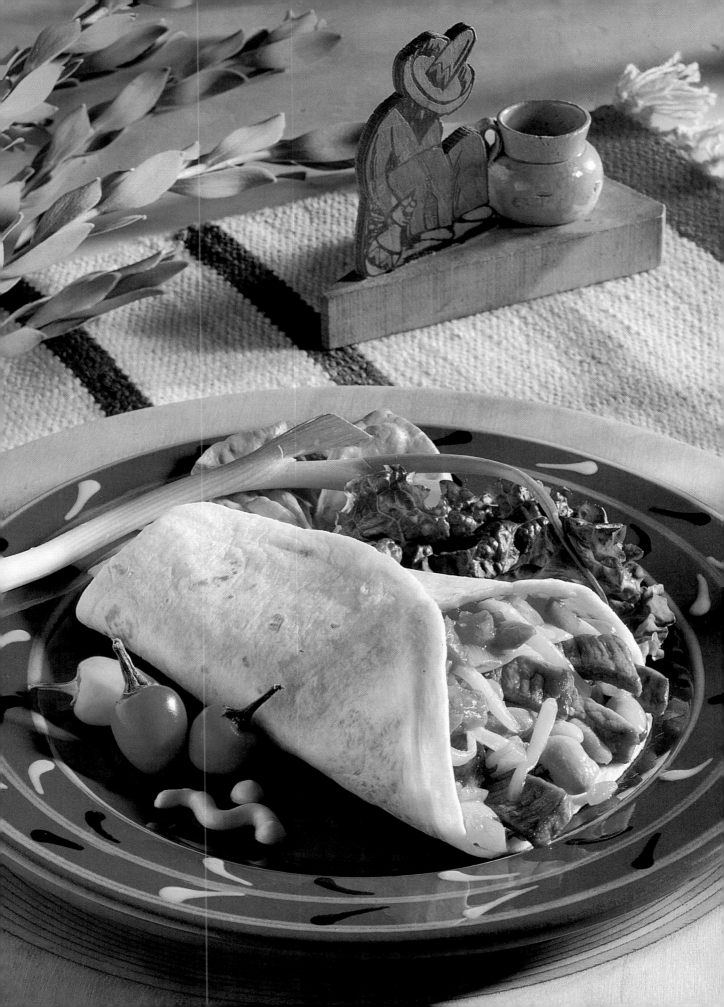

Desserts

Apple-Cherry Crisp

1 pound Granny Smith apples, peeled, cored and sliced ¼ inch thick
1 can (16 ounces) tart pie cherries packed in water, drained
1 can (16 ounces) dark sweet pitted cherries in heavy syrup, drained
2 teaspoons vanilla
1 teaspoon cinnamon
1 cup fruit-juice-sweetened granola without raisins*
⅓ cup sliced almonds
1 quart fat-free vanilla ice cream or frozen yogurt

1. Preheat oven to 350°F. Spray an 11×7-inch glass baking dish with nonstick cooking spray; set aside.

2. Combine apples, cherries, vanilla and cinnamon in large bowl; stir until well blended. Spoon into prepared baking dish. Cover with foil; bake 30 minutes.

3. Remove from oven; stir to distribute juices. Sprinkle granola and almonds evenly over fruit. Bake, uncovered, 15 minutes more or until juice is bubbling and almonds are golden; serve warm or at room temperature topped with ice cream. *Makes 8 servings*

*Available in the health food section of supermarkets.

Nutrients per Serving: Calories: 296 (15% Calories from Fat), Total Fat: 5 g, Saturated Fat: 2 g, Protein: 7 g, Carbohydrate: 59 g, Cholesterol: 0 mg, Sodium: 100 mg, Fiber: 3 g, Sugar: 28 g
Dietary Exchanges: 2 Starch/Bread, 2 Fruit, 1 Fat

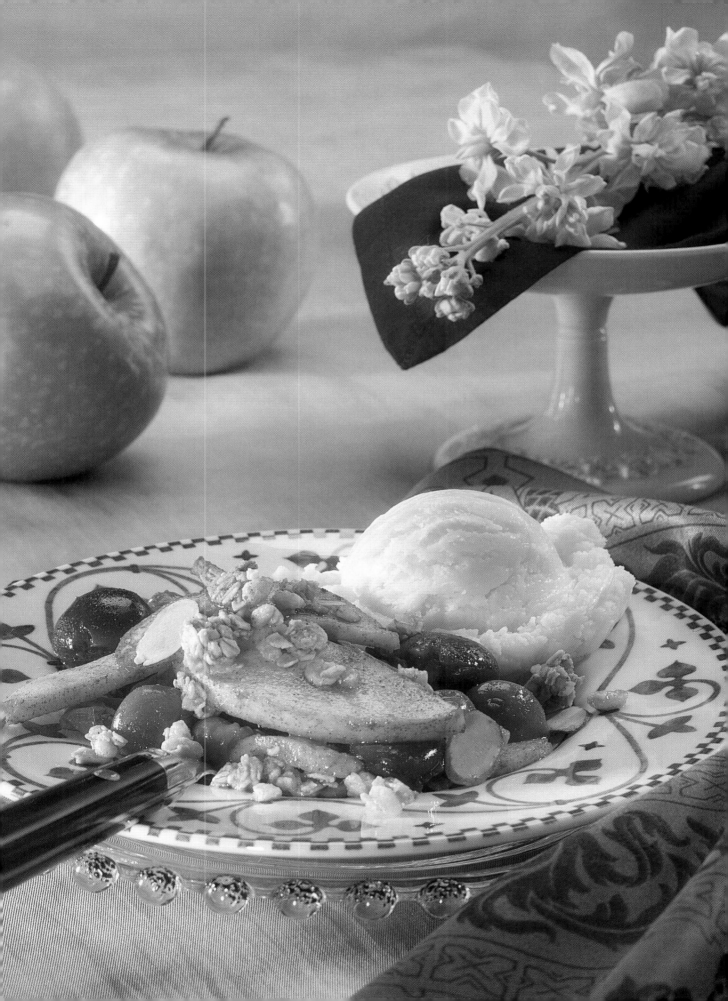

Mixed Berry Cheesecake

Crust:
- 1½ cups fruit-juice-sweetened breakfast cereal flakes*
- 15 dietetic butter-flavored cookies*
- 1 tablespoon vegetable oil

Cheesecake:
- 2 packages (8 ounces each) fat-free cream cheese, softened
- 2 cartons (8 ounces each) nonfat raspberry yogurt
- 1 package (8 ounces) Neufchâtel cream cheese, softened
- ½ cup all-fruit seedless blackberry preserves
- ½ cup all-fruit blueberry preserves
- 6 packages artificial sweetener *or* equivalent of ¼ cup sugar
- 1 tablespoon vanilla
- ¼ cup water
- 1 package (0.3 ounce) sugar-free strawberry-flavored gelatin

Topping:
- 3 cups fresh or frozen unsweetened mixed berries, thawed

*Available in the health food section of supermarkets.

1. Preheat oven to 400°F. Spray 10-inch springform pan with nonstick cooking spray.

2. To prepare crust, combine cereal, cookies and oil in food processor; process with on/off pulses until finely crushed. Press firmly onto bottom and ½ inch up side of pan. Bake 5 to 8 minutes or until crust is golden brown.

3. To prepare cheesecake, combine cream cheese, yogurt, Neufchâtel cheese, preserves, artificial sweetener and vanilla in large bowl. Beat with electric mixer at high speed until smooth.

4. Combine water and gelatin in small microwavable bowl; microwave at HIGH for 30 seconds to 1 minute or until water is boiling and gelatin is dissolved. Cool slightly. Add to cheese mixture; beat an additional 2 to 3 minutes or until well blended. Pour into springform pan; cover and refrigerate at least 24 hours. Top cheesecake with berries before serving.

Makes 12 servings

Nutrients per Serving: Calories: 248 (25% Calories from Fat), Total Fat: 7 g, Saturated Fat: 3 g, Protein: 10 g, Carbohydrate: 35 g, Cholesterol: 15 mg, Sodium: 386 mg, Fiber: 2 g, Sugar: 6 g
Dietary Exchanges: ½ Starch/Bread, 1 Lean Meat, 2 Fruit, ½ Fat

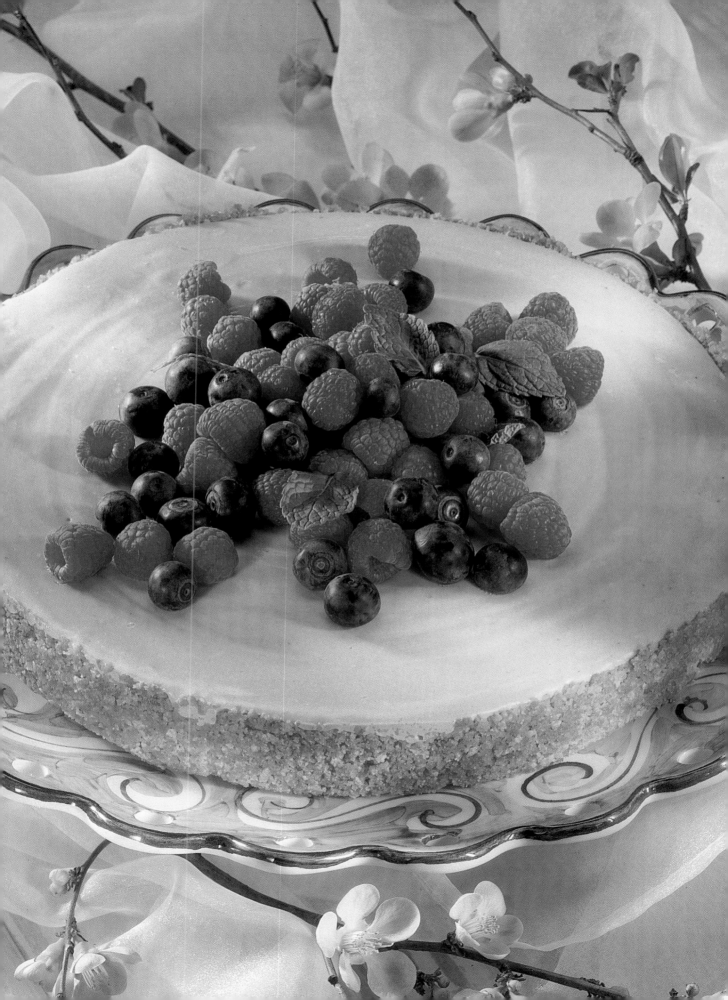

Key Lime Tarts

¾ **cup skim milk**
6 **tablespoons fresh lime juice**
2 **tablespoons cornstarch**
½ **cup cholesterol-free egg substitute**
½ **cup reduced-fat sour cream**
12 **packages artificial sweetener** *or* **equivalent of** ½ **cup sugar**
4 **sheets phyllo dough***
   Butter-flavored nonstick cooking spray
¾ **cup thawed fat-free nondairy whipped topping**

1. Whisk together milk, lime juice and cornstarch in medium saucepan. Cook over medium heat 2 to 3 minutes, stirring constantly until thick. Remove from heat.

2. Add egg substitute; whisk constantly for 30 seconds to allow egg substitute to cook. Stir in sour cream and artificial sweetener; cover and refrigerate until cool.

3. Preheat oven to 350°F. Spray 8 (2½-inch) muffin cups with cooking spray; set aside.

4. Place 1 sheet of phyllo dough on cutting board; spray with cooking spray. Top with second sheet of phyllo dough; spray with cooking spray. Top with third sheet of phyllo dough; spray with cooking spray. Top with last sheet; spray with cooking spray.

5. Cut stack of phyllo dough into 8 squares. Gently fit each stacked square into prepared muffin cups; press firmly against bottom and side. Bake 8 to 10 minutes or until golden brown. Carefully remove from muffin cups; cool on wire rack.

6. Divide lime mixture evenly among phyllo cups; top with whipped topping. Garnish with fresh raspberries and lime slices, if desired.

Makes 8 servings

*Cover with damp kitchen towel to prevent dough from drying out.

Nutrients per Serving: Calories: 82 (17% Calories from Fat), Total Fat: 1 g, Saturated Fat: trace, Protein: 3 g, Carbohydrate: 13 g, Cholesterol: 5 mg, Sodium: 88 mg, Fiber: trace, Sugar: 2 g
Dietary Exchanges: 1 Starch/Bread

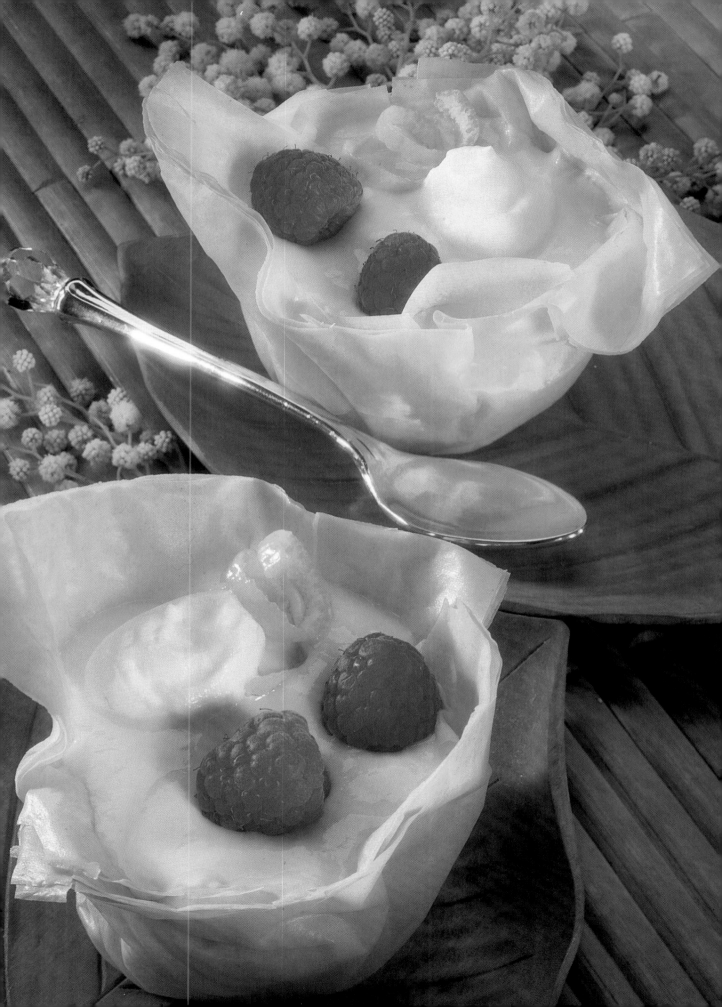

Chocolate-Strawberry Crêpes

Crêpes:
- ²/₃ **cup all-purpose flour**
- 2 **tablespoons unsweetened cocoa powder**
- 6 **packages artificial sweetener** *or* **equivalent of** ¼ **cup sugar**
- ¼ **teaspoon salt**
- 1¼ **cups skim milk**
- ½ **cup cholesterol-free egg substitute**
- 1 **tablespoon margarine, melted**
- 1 **teaspoon vanilla**
- **Nonstick cooking spray**

Filling and Topping:
- 4 **ounces fat-free cream cheese, softened**
- 1 **package (1.3 ounces) chocolate-fudge-flavored sugar-free instant pudding mix**
- 1½ **cups skim milk**
- ¼ **cup all-fruit strawberry preserves**
- 2 **tablespoons water**
- 2 **cups fresh hulled and quartered strawberries**

1. To prepare crêpes, combine flour, cocoa, artificial sweetener and salt in food processor; process to blend. Add milk, egg substitute, margarine and vanilla; process until smooth. Let stand at room temperature 30 minutes.

2. Spray 7-inch nonstick skillet with cooking spray; heat over medium-high heat. Pour 2 tablespoons crêpe batter into hot pan. Immediately rotate pan back and forth to swirl batter over entire surface of pan. Cook 1 to 2 minutes or until crêpe is brown around edge and top is dry. Carefully turn crêpe with spatula and cook 30 seconds more. Transfer crêpe to waxed paper to cool. Repeat with remaining batter, spraying pan with cooking spray as needed. Separate crêpes with sheets of waxed paper.

3. To prepare chocolate filling, beat cream cheese in medium bowl with electric mixer at high speed until smooth; set aside. Prepare chocolate pudding with skim milk according to package directions. Gradually add pudding to cream cheese mixture; beat at high speed for 3 minutes.

4. To prepare strawberry topping, combine preserves and water in large bowl until smooth. Add strawberries; toss to coat.

5. Spread 2 tablespoons chocolate filling evenly over surface of crêpe; roll tightly. Repeat with remaining crêpes. Place two crêpes on each plate. Spoon ¼ cup strawberry topping over each serving. Serve immediately.

Makes 8 servings (2 crêpes each)

Nutrients per Serving: Calories: 161 (13% Calories from Fat), Total Fat: 2 g, Saturated Fat: trace, Protein: 8 g, Carbohydrate: 27 g, Cholesterol: 1 mg, Sodium: 374 mg, Fiber: 1 g, Sugar: 6 g
Dietary Exchanges: 1 Lean Meat, 2 Fruit

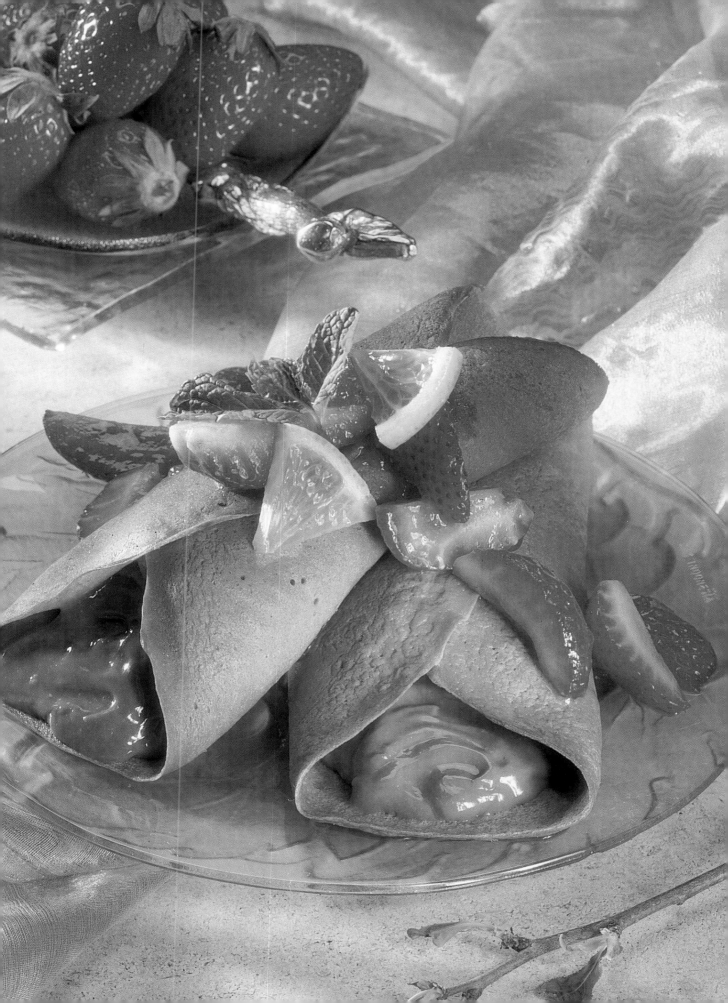

Lemon Raspberry Tiramisu

Tiramisu, which literally means "pick me up," is a popular Italian dessert. This variation, which features raspberries rather than coffee and chocolate, is the perfect ending to a special meal.

2 packages (8 ounces each) fat-free cream cheese, softened
6 packages artificial sweetener *or* equivalent of ¼ cup sugar
1 teaspoon vanilla
⅓ cup water
1 package (0.3 ounce) sugar-free lemon-flavored gelatin
2 cups thawed fat-free nondairy whipped topping
½ cup all-fruit red raspberry preserves
¼ cup water
2 tablespoons marsala wine
2 packages (3 ounces each) ladyfingers
1 pint fresh raspberries or frozen unsweetened raspberries, thawed

1. Combine cream cheese, artificial sweetener and vanilla in large bowl. Beat with electric mixer at high speed until smooth; set aside.

2. Combine water and gelatin in small microwavable bowl; microwave at HIGH 30 seconds to 1 minute or until water is boiling and gelatin is dissolved. Cool slightly.

3. Add gelatin mixture to cheese mixture; beat 1 minute. Add whipped topping; beat 1 minute more, scraping sides of bowl. Set aside.

4. Whisk together preserves, water and marsala in small bowl until well blended. Reserve 2 tablespoons of preserves mixture; set aside. Spread ⅓ cup of preserves mixture evenly over bottom of 11×7-inch glass baking dish.

5. Split ladyfingers in half; place half in bottom of baking dish. Spread ½ of cheese mixture evenly over ladyfingers; sprinkle 1 cup of raspberries evenly over cheese mixture. Top with remaining ladyfingers; spread remaining preserves mixture over ladyfingers. Top with remaining cheese mixture. Cover; refrigerate for at least 2 hours. Sprinkle with remaining raspberries and drizzle with reserved 2 tablespoons of preserves mixture before serving.   *Makes 12 servings*

Nutrients per Serving: Calories: 158 (9% Calories from Fat), Total Fat: 1 g, Saturated Fat: trace, Protein: 7 g, Carbohydrate: 26 g, Cholesterol: 52 mg, Sodium: 272 mg, Fiber: 1 g, Sugar: 3 g
Dietary Exchanges: 2 Starch/Bread

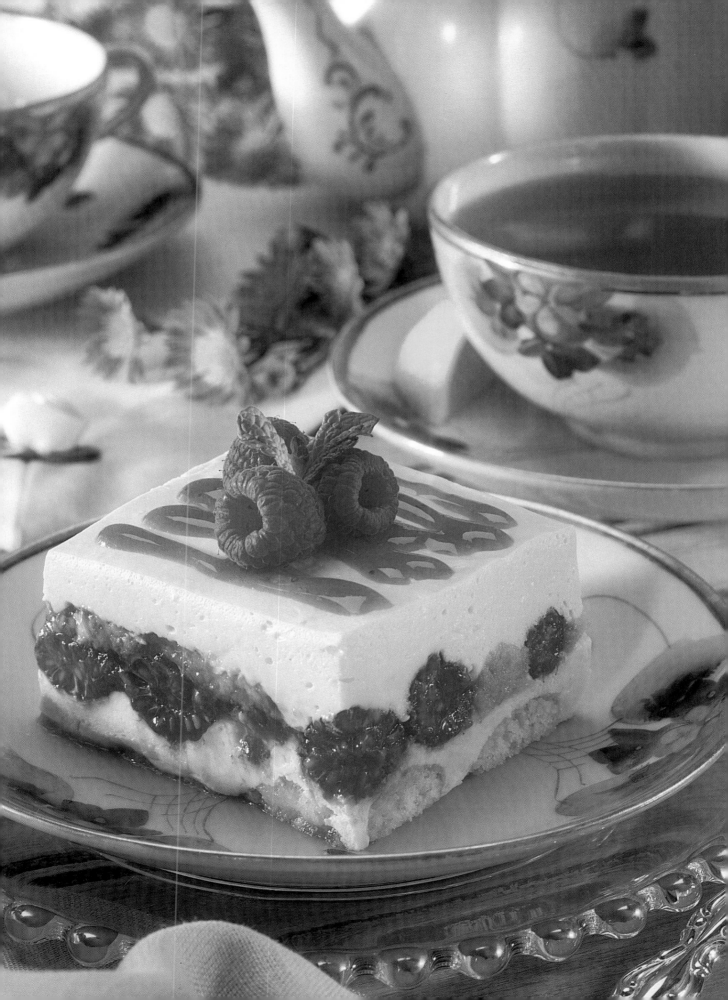

Tropical Bread Pudding with Piña Colada Sauce

Bread Pudding:
>   6 cups cubed day-old French bread
>   1 cup skim milk
>   1 cup frozen orange-pineapple-banana juice concentrate, thawed
>   ½ cup cholesterol-free egg substitute
>   2 teaspoons vanilla
>   ½ teaspoon butter-flavored extract
>   1 can (8 ounces) crushed pineapple in juice, undrained
>   ½ cup golden raisins

Piña Colada Sauce:
>   ¾ cup all-fruit pineapple preserves
>   ⅓ cup shredded unsweetened coconut, toasted
>   1 teaspoon rum *or* ⅛ teaspoon rum extract

1. To prepare bread pudding, preheat oven to 350°F. Spray 11×7-inch glass baking dish with nonstick cooking spray. Place cubed bread in large bowl; set aside.

2. Combine milk, juice concentrate, egg substitute, vanilla and butter-flavored extract in another large bowl; mix until smooth. Drain pineapple; reserve juice. Add milk mixture, pineapple and raisins to bread; gently mix with large spoon. Spoon bread mixture evenly into prepared baking dish and flatten slightly; bake, uncovered, 40 minutes. Cool slightly.

3. To prepare Piña Colada Sauce, add water to reserved pineapple juice to equal ¼ cup. Combine juice, preserves, coconut and rum in microwavable bowl. Microwave at HIGH 2 to 3 minutes or until sauce is hot and bubbling; cool to room temperature.

4. Divide pudding among 8 plates; top each serving with 2 tablespoons of Piña Colada Sauce.   *Makes 8 servings*

Nutrients per Serving: Calories: 280 (6% Calories from Fat), Total Fat: 2 g, Saturated Fat: 1 g, Protein: 6 g, Carbohydrate: 61 g, Cholesterol: 1 mg, Sodium: 178 mg, Fiber: 1 g, Sugar: 12 g
Dietary Exchanges: 1 Starch/Bread, 3 Fruit, ½ Fat

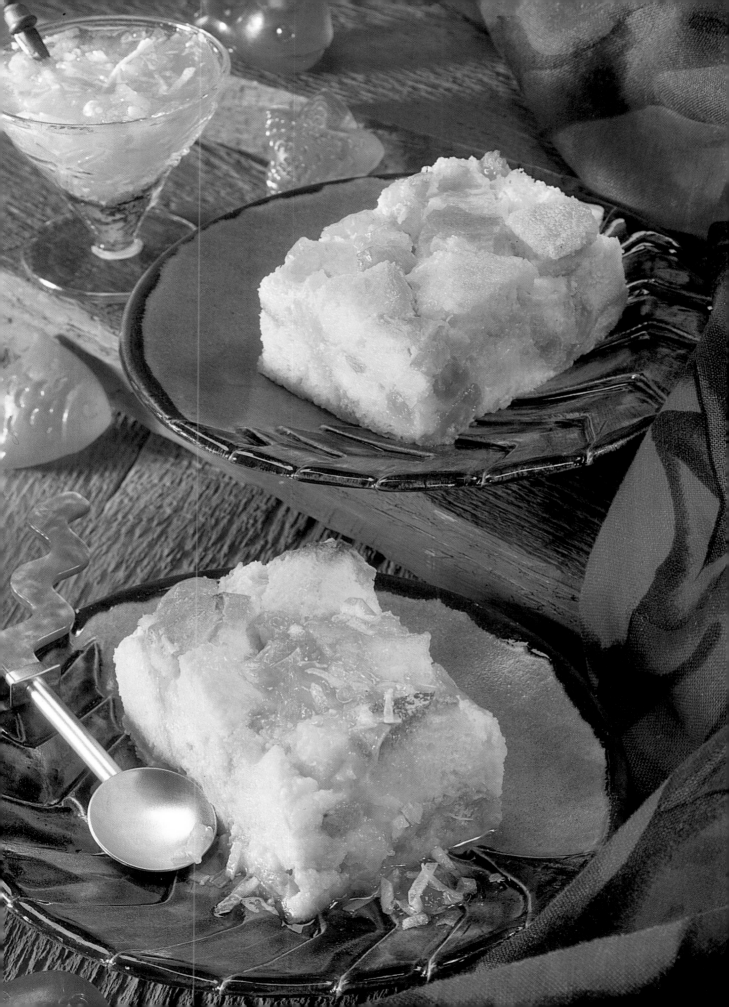

METRIC CONVERSION CHART

VOLUME MEASUREMENTS (dry)

1/8 teaspoon = 0.5 mL
1/4 teaspoon = 1 mL
1/2 teaspoon = 2 mL
3/4 teaspoon = 4 mL
1 teaspoon = 5 mL
1 tablespoon = 15 mL
2 tablespoons = 30 mL
1/4 cup = 60 mL
1/3 cup = 75 mL
1/2 cup = 125 mL
2/3 cup = 150 mL
3/4 cup = 175 mL
1 cup = 250 mL
2 cups = 1 pint = 500 mL
3 cups = 750 mL
4 cups = 1 quart = 1 L

VOLUME MEASUREMENTS (fluid)

1 fluid ounce (2 tablespoons) = 30 mL
4 fluid ounces (1/2 cup) = 125 mL
8 fluid ounces (1 cup) = 250 mL
12 fluid ounces (1 1/2 cups) = 375 mL
16 fluid ounces (2 cups) = 500 mL

WEIGHTS (mass)

1/2 ounce = 15 g
1 ounce = 30 g
3 ounces = 90 g
4 ounces = 120 g
8 ounces = 225 g
10 ounces = 285 g
12 ounces = 360 g
16 ounces = 1 pound = 450 g

DIMENSIONS

1/16 inch = 2 mm
1/8 inch = 3 mm
1/4 inch = 6 mm
1/2 inch = 1.5 cm
3/4 inch = 2 cm
1 inch = 2.5 cm

OVEN TEMPERATURES

250°F = 120°C
275°F = 140°C
300°F = 150°C
325°F = 160°C
350°F = 180°C
375°F = 190°C
400°F = 200°C
425°F = 220°C
450°F = 230°C

BAKING PAN SIZES

Utensil	Size in Inches/Quarts	Metric Volume	Size in Centimeters
Baking or Cake Pan (square or rectangular)	8×8×2	2 L	20×20×5
	9×9×2	2.5 L	23×23×5
	12×8×2	3 L	30×20×5
	13×9×2	3.5 L	33×23×5
Loaf Pan	8×4×3	1.5 L	20×10×7
	9×5×3	2 L	23×13×7
Round Layer Cake Pan	8×1½	1.2 L	20×4
	9×1½	1.5 L	23×4
Pie Plate	8×1¼	750 mL	20×3
	9×1¼	1 L	23×3
Baking Dish or Casserole	1 quart	1 L	—
	1½ quart	1.5 L	—
	2 quart	2 L	—